Alan J. Smith, Ph.D.

Springer Series on Medical Education

SERIES EDITOR: Steven Jonas, M.D.

VOLUME 1 Problem-Based Learning: An Approach to Medical Education
Howard S. Barrows, M.D., and Robyn M. Tamblyn, B.Sc.N.

VOLUME 2 The Evaluation of Teaching in Medical Schools
Robert M. Rippey, Ph.D.

VOLUME 3 The Art of Teaching Primary Care
Archie S. Golden, M.D. M.P.H., Dennis G. Carlson, M.D., M.P.H., M.A., and Jan L. Hagen, M.S.W., *Editors*

VOLUME 4 Medical Education in the Ambulatory Setting: An Evaluation
Loyd J. Wollstadt, M.D., Sc.M., Dennis A. Frate, Ph.D., and Mark G. Meyer, M.A.T.

VOLUME 5 Teaching Preventive Medicine in Primary Care
William H. Barker, M.D.

VOLUME 6 The Interpersonal Dimension in Medical Education
Agnes G. Rezler, Ph.D., and Joseph A. Flaherty, M.D.

VOLUME 7 Assessing Clinical Competence
Victor R. Neufeld, M.D., FRCP (C), and Geoffrey R. Norman, Ph.D., *Editors*

VOLUME 8 How to Design a Problem-Based Curriculum for the Preclinical Years
Howard S. Barrows, M.D., FRCP (C)

VOLUME 9 Implementing Problem-Based Medical Education: Lessons from Successful Innovations
Arthur Kaufman, M.D., *Editor*

VOLUME 10 Clinical Teaching for Medical Residents: Roles, Techniques, and Programs
Janine C. Edwards, Ph.D., and Robert L. Marier, M.D., FACP, *Editors*

VOLUME 11 A Practical Guide to Clinical Teaching in Medicine
Kaaren C. Douglas, M.D., M.S.P.H., Michael C. Hosokawa, Ed.D., and Frank H. Lawler, M.D., M.S.P.H.

VOLUME 12 Successful Faculty in Academic Medicine: Essential Skills and How to Acquire Them
Carole J. Bland, Ph.D., Constance C. Schmitz, M.A., Frank T. Stritter, Ph.D., Rebecca C. Henry, Ph.D., and John J. Aluise, Ph.D.

VOLUME 13 Innovation in Medical Education: An Evaluation of Its Present Status
Zohair M. Nooman, Henk G. Schmidt, and Esmat S. Ezzat, *Editors*

VOLUME 14 The Politics of Reform in Medical Education and Health Services: The Negev Project
Basil Porter, M.B.B.Ch., M.P.H., and William E. Seidelman, M.D.

VOLUME 15 Medical Teaching in Ambulatory Care: A Practical Guide
Warren Rubenstein, M.D., and Yves Talbot, M.D.

VOLUME 16 Collaborative Clinical Education: The Foundation of Effective Health Care
Jane Westberg, Ph.D., Hilliard Jason, M.D.

VOLUME 17 Assessment Measures in Medical School, Residency, and Practice: The Connections
Joseph S. Gonnella, M.D., Mohammadreza Hojat, Ph.D., James B. Erdmann, Ph.D., and J. Jon Veloski, M.S.

Joseph S. Gonnella, M.D., Senior Vice President for Academic Affairs and Dean of Jefferson Medical College, Thomas Jefferson University. Dr. Gonnella is responsible for the development and management of the administrative affairs and academic programs of education, research, and patient care in the Medical College, and is also a Professor of Medicine. He is the founder and Director of the Medical College's Center for Research in Medical Education and Health Care. He received his B.A. from Dartmouth College, *summa cum laude*, and his M.D. from Harvard Medical School. He has been awarded the Commendatore nell Ordine from the President of Italy, the Dongbaeg Medal from the President of Korea, and the Presidential Medal from Dartmouth College. He is currently a member of the Liaison Committee on Medical Education, the body responsible for the accreditation of all medical schools in the United States and Canada.

Mohammadreza Hojat, Ph.D., is Director of the Jefferson Longitudinal Study of Medical Students and Graduates, and Research Associate Professor of Psychiatry and Human Behavior at Jefferson Medical College. He received his Ph.D. from the University of Pennsylvania. Dr. Hojat is a licensed psychologist and in addition to medical education, other areas of his research interest include noncognitive factors in academic achievement, early mother–child attachment and personality development, and dynamics of loneliness experiences. He has served as a co-editor (with Dr. Rick Crandall) of a book on loneliness. Dr. Hojat has published extensively, and contributed more than 70 articles to professional journals on educational, psychological, and social issues. He is listed in *Who's Who Among Human Services Professionals.*

James B. Erdmann, Ph.D., is the Associate Dean for Administration and Registrar, and Professor, Department of Medicine, Jefferson Medical College, Thomas Jefferson University. Prior to his current position, Dr. Erdmann served for 17 years as Director of the Division of Educational Measurement and Research at the Association of American Medical Colleges (AAMC), where he was responsible for the development and conduct of the Medical College Admission Test program; research on admissions issues, the conduct of the AAMC's 20-year follow-up of 2,800 medical school graduates of the Class of 1960; and research and development of student clinical evaluation systems for U.S. medical schools. He has published articles on techniques for the assessment of the problem-solving process in medicine and in more general contexts. Dr. Erdmann has served on several editorial boards and is listed in the *Dictionary of International Biography, Who's Who in the World, Men and Women in Science, Who's Who in Health Care,* and *Leaders in Education.*

J. Jon Veloski, M.S., is Director of Medical Educational Research at the Center for Research in Medical Education and Health Care, Jefferson Medical College, Thomas Jefferson University. He is especially interested in the development of methods for evaluation of clinical competence. He played a leadership role in several studies of the relationship between performance in medical school and supervisors' ratings of clinical competence after graduation. Currently Mr. Veloski serves as co-investigator of a 5-year project funded by the American Board of Family Practice to develop assessment measures of clinical competence of family physicians, and is co-project director of a study funded by the Health Resources Services Administration on the relationship between the characteristics of medical schools and their output of primary care physicians.

ASSESSMENT MEASURES IN MEDICAL SCHOOL, RESIDENCY, AND PRACTICE

The Connections

Joseph S. Gonnella, MD
Mohammadreza Hojat, PhD
James B. Erdmann, PhD
J. Jon Veloski, MS
Editors

SPRINGER PUBLISHING COMPANY
New York

Springer Publishing Company, Inc.
536 Broadway
New York, NY 10012

93 94 95 96 97 / 5 4 3 2 1

Library of Congress Cataloging-in-Publication Data

Assessment measures in medical school, residency, and practice: The connections / Joseph S. Gonnella . . . [et al.], editors.
p. cm. — (Springer series on medical education; v. 17)
Originally published as a special issue to the journal, *Academic medicine*. Includes bibliographical references and index.
ISBN 0–8261–8350–6
1. Medical education—United States—Evaluation. 2. Clinical competence—United States. I. Gonnella, Joseph S. II. Academic medicine. III. Series.
[DNLM: 1. Education, Medical. 2. Competency-Based Education. 3. Professional Competence. W1 SP685SE v. 17 1993 / W 18 A8345 1993]
R745.A74 1993
610'.71'173—dc20
DNLM/DLC
for Library of Congress 93-35462
CIP

Printed in the United States of America

Cover and interior design by Holly Block
Cover illustration by Dan Kuetemeyer

To our wives

J. S. G.
M. H.
J. B. E.
J. J. V.

Contents

Part III: Empirical Findings

Part IV: Epilogue

Contributors

Dominic Albo, Jr., MD, Associate Professor of Surgery and Associate Dean for Clinical Affairs, Department of Surgery, School of Medicine, University of Utah, Salt Lake City.

Louise Arnold, PhD, Assistant Dean, Office of Medical Education and Research, School of Medicine, University of Missouri–Kansas City.

Bingxun Liu, MD, Former Director, Department of Medical Education, Ministry of Public Health, People's Republic of China.

Charles Boelen, MD, DPH, MSc, Chief Medical Officer for Educational Development of Human Resources for Health, Division of Development of Human Resources for Health, World Health Organization, Geneva, Switzerland.

Susan M. Case, PhD, Senior Evaluation Officer and Exam System Coordinator, Step 2, National Board of Medical Examiners, Philadelphia, PA.

Jerry A. Colliver, PhD, Professor and Director, Division of Statistics Research Consulting, School of Medicine, Southern Illinois University, Springfield.

Linda H. Distlehorst, PhD, Assistant Dean for Curricular Affairs and Assistant Professor, Department of Medical Education, School of Medicine, Southern Illinois University, Springfield.

Ruth-Marie E. Fincher, MD, Associate Professor of Medicine and Associate Dean for Curriculum, School of Medicine, The Medical College of Georgia, Augusta.

Ute Fuchs, Dr.Med.Habil., Lecturer, Department of Obstetrics and Gynecology, University of Tuebingen, Tuebingen, Germany.

Eugene A. Hildreth, MD, MACP, Immediate Past President of the American College of Physicians and Clinical Professor of Medicine at the University of Pennsylvania Reading Hospital and Medical Center, Reading, PA.

Susan Howell, MSS, Coordinator, Outcomes Projects, Center for Research in Medical Education and Health Care, Jefferson Medical College, Thomas Jefferson University, Philadelphia, PA.

Donald G. Kassebaum, MD, Vice President, Division of Educational Research and Assessment, Association of American Medical Colleges, Washington, DC.

Terrance T. Kuske, MD, Professor of Medicine, School of Medicine, Medical College of Georgia, Augusta.

Lloyd A. Lewis, PhD, Professor, Medical Education, School of Medicine, Medical College of Georgia, Augusta.

David M. Macfadyen, MBchB, MSc, FRCP Edin., Director, Program Management, World Health Organization, Copenhagen, Denmark.

Ronald J. Markert, PhD, Professor, Department of Medicine, School of Medicine, Wright State University, Dayton, Ohio.

Leona E. Markson, ScD, Associate Director, Clinical Outcomes Research, Research Assistant, Professor of Medicine, Center for Research in Medical Education and Health Care, Jefferson Medical College, Thomas Jefferson University, Philadelphia, PA.

Jack Marshall, MD, Director of CHECK Program; Director of Resource Development Family Medicine Program and Senior Examiner, The Royal Australian College of General Practitioners (RACGP), North Adelaide, South Australia.

Christine McGuire, Emerita Professor of Medical Education, University of Illinois College of Medicine, Chicago.

George E. Miller, MD, Emeritus Professor of Medical Education, University of Illinois College of Medicine, Chicago.

David B. Nash, MD, MBA, Director of Health Policy and Clinical Outcomes, Jefferson Medical College and Thomas Jefferson University Hospital, Thomas Jefferson University, Philadelphia, PA.

Hans E. Renschler, Dr.Med., Professor Emeritus of Medical Education, University of Bonn, Bonn, Germany.

Horacio J. A. Rimoldi, MD, PhD, Editor of *Interdisciplinaria*; Director CIIPME, Buenos Aires, Argentina.

David B. Swanson, PhD, Senior Evaluation Officer and Exam System Coordinator, Step 1, National Board of Medical Examiners, Philadelphia, PA.

Calvin W. Taylor, PhD, Research Professor in Creativity and Wellness, University of Utah, Salt Lake City.

Steven J. Verhulst, PhD, Assistant Professor, Division of Statistics and Research Consulting, School of Medicine, Southern Illinois University, Springfield.

Wolfgang H. Vogel, PhD, Professor, Department of Pharmacology, Jefferson Medical College, Thomas Jefferson University, Philadelphia, PA.

Nu V. Vu, PhD, Professor, Department of Medical Education, School of Medicine, Southern Illinois University, Springfield.

T. Lee Willoughby, MS, Director, Computer and Evaluation Resources, School of Medicine, University of Missouri–Kansas City.

Foreword to the Expanded Edition

In 1966, as a Fellow in Medical Education at the University of Illinois, Joseph S. Gonnella selected as his research project a study entitled, "Clinical Instruction and Patient Care." The final report of that work opened with these words: "The ultimate criterion of educational effectiveness in medicine is the quality of care rendered to patients." That interest in the educational input/performance outcome relationship has now endured for more than a quarter century. It has been a central feature of the landmark longitudinal study he and his associates at the Jefferson Medical College Center for Research in Medical Education and Health Care have conducted over the last decade. *Assessment Measures in Medical School, Residency, and Practice: The Connections* is a natural outcome of that work, here supplemented and complemented with studies by colleagues at home and abroad who have had similar concerns.

Conventional wisdom would tell us that the best predictor of future performance is past performance. However, it has been difficult to identify a consistent relationship between the academic measures of medical student achievement and the professional behavior of residents and practitioners. Positive correlations, when found, are commonly so weak as to be unconvincing; and the infrequency of even weak correlations between basic medical science grades and clinical performance has often led to strong criticism of science courses which appear to have so little relevance to the objectives of medical education.

Faculty members must occasionally be reminded (as Wolfgang Vogel does here) that relevance, like beauty, is usually in the eye of the beholder. What is taught, and what is tested, seems more often to reflect the interests of teachers than the needs of learners. This inescapable truth seems at the heart of the problem reflected in our unending search for a "core curriculum" whose segments will both satisfy all the players, and correlate highly with the quality of care delivered by medical school graduates.

This passionate concern for curriculum content, the science of medicine, too often ignores the social, economic and cultural realities that equally influence the nature of health care. It is these factors probably far more than what is now taught and evaluated in medical school which determine the form of health services. And if that is true we should not be surprised that basic science grades, even clinical science ratings, do not exhibit strong relationships with measures of physician performance. As the editors point out in their penultimate paragraph, ". . . we could tinker with the medical school component forever and see little impact on patient outcomes."

In the continuum of medical education the nature of teaching, learning, and assessment undergoes a steady change from an early focus upon acquisition of knowledge, to a midstream preoccupation with competence, and an ultimate concern for performance. While these qualities surely overlap they are by no means identical. As Arnold and Willoughby (chapter 7) wisely point out, it is possible that relationships between findings at these several stages of education are inherently limited because the performance expected of residents may not be mere extensions of those expected of medical students.

This should not imply that what goes on in the medical school is unrelated to professional performance outcomes. With few exceptions, the empirical studies reported here appear to support the conventional wisdom, at least when academic and performance measurements are similar. The trouble begins with extrapolation from the assessment of one characteristic to conclusions about another, with lumping data derived from different sources at different times using implicit criteria (or even those that are explicit) into some global description of achievement, with the acceptance of numerical ratings as accurate descriptions of what students or graduates actually do. Even the most elegant statistical manipulation of such findings cannot easily be translated into behavioral significance.

The message this book delivers most forcefully, and most persuasively, is that we need to be more careful in the design of studies that attempt to explore relationships between medical school instruction and subsequent independent clinical behavior, and in the generalizations we draw from these findings. But it is not these cautionary statements alone that should influence future investigators. The principles and practices enunciated so clearly in the background papers (chapters 1 and 2) and the Epilogue could set the stage for a new generation of studies that will be even more informative than those that have gone before.

And that is, after all, the way in which science, behavioral or biological, makes progress.

GEORGE E. MILLER, M.D.

Foreword to the Original Edition

The measure of success is the result. This is not news, although in a world of educational jargon like "outcomes assessment" it may be necessary to remind ourselves that the most elementary way to assess the outcomes of teaching and learning is to examine the students. But mastery of first principles in biochemistry is one thing, and command of the skills and behaviors for medical practice is something else.

Despite this obvious dichotomy, educators continue to look for a correlation between students' performances in medical school and the behavior of graduates during residency training and practice. Indeed, it starts even earlier, as admission committees try to predict educability and future professional conduct (they are better at the former than the latter) on the basis of premedical school grades and scores on the Medical College Admission Test (MCAT). While it might be argued, as is done by Christine McGuire in this monograph, that these predictors account for only a small fraction of the variance in grades in basic science courses, the strength of the signals consistently predicting 97% graduation rates (89% for African Americans) covers up most of the noise in the system (to borrow a metaphor from Gonnella et al.). For that matter, the singularly most powerful predictor of success in medical practice is admission to medical school.

If we were recruiting for the NBA instead of for residency programs, we would give scant attention to college grades in English composition and American history and would look instead at performance on passing, shooting, running, and learning and executing maneuvers for defense and scoring. We would find better basketball players that way, and we also would avoid the flaws that arise when predictor and criterion variables are not aligned.

While the proficiency achieved by a college basketball player is largely the product of coaching and training outside the regular program of undergraduate education, the preparation for medical practice is mostly the result of teaching within the curriculum. So it stands to reason that there ought to be inklings along the educational continuum about a medical student's future capability.

The editors of this monograph have collected an assortment of perspectives and empirical findings on the connections between assessment measures in medical school, residency, and practice. A number of studies show relationships between measures in medical school and after graduation, and these are stacked up against the extensive literature to the contrary. In the Background section, McGuire and Gonnella et al. interpret the differences and enumerate the conceptual and methodological factors that uncouple the measures of achievement in medical school from performance after graduation.

Of course, without establishing performance criteria in practice it is not possible to find, let alone measure, the behavioral parameters at discrete points along the continuum of medical education that might predict future conduct. Contributors to this monograph give various views of physician competence in practice and describe some of the correlations with assessments during medical school. Not surprisingly, the associations are stronger when there is greater identity between the formative behaviors that are measured and the criterion elements of later practice. But even this congruence cannot overcome the contamination by intervening experiences when predictor and criterion variables are measured too far apart.

A lot of work has gone into studies that try to link performance as a physician with diverse measures taken during medical students' formative years. The pattern of correlations between knowledge tests during and after medical school has given support to the use of the National Board of Medical Examiners' (NBME's) examinations in the selection of residents. Case et al., in this monograph, cast light on the relationship between NBME examination scores and performances on several of the specialty board examinations, while acknowledging the importance of many other traits not measured by written tests in predicting success in residency training.

In too many instances, however, efforts to draw correlations between later clinical competencies and proxies like antecedent grade averages and NBME examination scores strain credulity as well as the limits of Pearson product-moment correlation techniques. One is reminded of the attempts of yesterday to estimate the grade of aortic stenosis by studying the contour of the brachial artery pressure pulse. Just as pulse analysis gave way to the direct imaging of the aortic valve, so now we are able to evaluate clinical ability directly as it is taking form. Vu et al.

describe the usefulness of students' performances on standardized-patient-based postclerkship examinations as a predictor of first-year residency supervisors' ratings.

With this monograph, the editors shed a new light of rationality on the association between assessment measures during medical school and after graduation. Not surprisingly, the most convincing work comes from their own Jefferson longitudinal study of medical students and graduates, the paragon assessment of educational outcomes.

Some of these reports will be of considerable help to the educational stewardship of every medical school. Present-day political and social accountability calls for something more than a declarative judgment that the content and process of medical education yield graduate physicians with exemplary professional skills and behavior. As a condition of accreditation, medical schools must show that they have a system to evaluate the extent to which their educational objectives are achieved. And schools undertaking innovative educational programs will need a method of evaluating the results that goes beyond mastery of individual courses.

Hojat et al. draw two important conclusions that deserve underscoring: that medical school faculty members should have confidence that their judgments are valid; and that more attention ought to be paid to students at the lower end of the performance spectrum, who should be required to correct their deficiencies before they graduate, because their future performance is likely to be a reflection of their past showing. These authors also provide some important advice to residency program directors about paying attention to the performance dimensions that are more relevant to their own objectives.

Dr. William Osler never heard of Pearson *r*, but he had it right when he observed: "As one watches a man handle a patient it is easy to tell whether or not he has had a proper training, and for this purpose fifteen minutes at the bedside are worth three hours at the desk."

Donald G. Kassebaum, M.D.
Vice President for Educational Research
and Assessment
Association of American Medical Colleges

Acknowledgments

This volume represents the efforts of many contributors in addition to the authors of the articles. Addeane Caelleigh, the editor of *Academic Medicine,* encouraged us to assemble the monograph and provided us with invaluable guidance and suggestions throughout this endeavor. Her contribution, as well as the support of the AAMC, provided the forum to present the work of those at the forefront of medical education research and training. In addition, other editors at *Academic Medicine* —Albert Bradford, Christopher Greene, and Philip Diamond contributed valuable critiques and revisions to the manuscripts, and Sandra Lovegrove of Hanley and Belfus, Inc., skillfully oversaw the final editing and technical production of the original publication of the monograph.

The following invited reviewers made important contributions to the quality of the monograph by providing extensive comments and suggestions to the authors: Mark A. Albanese, Ph.D., University of Iowa College of Medicine; Louise Arnold, Ph.D., University of Missouri–Kansas City School of Medicine; James J. Diamond, Ph.D., Jefferson Medical College of Thomas Jefferson University; Charles P. Friedman, Ph.D., University of North Carolina at Chapel Hill School of Medicine; John J. Norcini, Ph.D., the American Board of Internal Medicine; William C. McGaghie, Ph.D., Northwestern University Medical School, and David B. Swanson, Ph.D., the National Board of Medical Examiners. We would also like to acknowledge the comments and evaluations made by an anonymous reviewer provided by *Academic Medicine.* We thank Dr. James J. Diamond, Dr. Sylvia Fields, and Christine McGuire for their constructive comments on our articles. Janet Hoefling and Robert Hallisey prepared the figures for our papers. Deep appreciation is also extended to Diane Pohl for her editorial assistance and to Maryann Zippel for her exceptional secretarial skills. We gratefully acknowledge the permission by the Association of American Medical Colleges to reproduce the entire copyrighted materials of the

February 1993 supplement to *Academic Medicine* in the present volume. And finally we would like to thank Mary Grace Luke, Senior Acquisitions Editor, and Pam Ritzer of the Springer Publishing Company for their valuable efforts in the publication of this expanded edition.

Joseph S. Gonnella, M.D.
Mohammadreza Hojat, Ph.D.
James B. Erdmann, Ph.D.
J. Jon Veloski, M.S.

Jefferson Medical College
Philadelphia, Pennsylvania

Introduction: Embarking on a Journey

This monograph documents an early stage of what may be likened to a journey—a quest to capture the essence of the relationship between performance in the controlled environment of medical school and performance in the uncontrolled world of practice after graduation. We invite our readers to join us in exploring the terrain of this heretofore vague relationship, with the guidance offered by the experts who have contributed to the monograph.

Our journey gained its initial momentum long before we and our contemporaries took to the high road of medical education. It is a logical extension of the debate over the relevance of medical education to the practice of medicine that has raged for decades. This ongoing controversy gains renewed vigor whenever the curriculum is scrutinized and reform is advocated. Inevitably the cry is heard that the basic sciences are irrelevant to clinical medicine. Those making the noise are typically to be found running Pearson product moment correlations between academic performance in medical school (usually in the first two years) and some measure of performance as a physician—a low or nonsignificant correlation sparks a quick conclusion that performance in the academic setting is irrelevant. Occasionally a review of the literature leads to a similar judgment.

On the other hand, there are those of us who feel that the system is supported by compelling logic and believe that the issue needs to be examined in greater depth. Not to do so implies that the question is not worth asking. It implies that the "Function and Structure of a Medical School," our accreditation standard, is a fiction created to justify the status quo, a delusion that we should not perpetuate. Failure to explore the issue suggests that we may be afraid to discover the answer because our real motivation is to protect our schools and our current way of life.

Government is increasingly mandating accountability, and this emphasis has permeated the field of testing, where government has already demanded that selection tests be shown predictive of relevant criterion behavior. Outcome assessment is also in vogue, and it is important in many educational settings now to require evaluation of outcomes to justify educational investments. The lack of a relationship between educational outcomes and process measurements is certainly counter to the trend.

For these reasons, and more, the authors saw value in addressing the nature of the relationship between performances before and after graduation from medical school.

Academic Medicine, the official journal of the Association of American Medical Colleges, seemed to be the best forum for our efforts because of its purpose to serve the academic medicine community and because of its knowledgeable readers, who have a vested interest in the issue. Addeane Calleigh, the editor of *Academic Medicine*, was receptive to the idea and suggested this special monograph, which was originally published as a special supplement to *Academic Medicine* (Volume 68, Number 2, February 1993 Supplement).

We prepared an action plan, a timetable, and a proposed table of contents. A call for papers was published in the November 1991 issue of *Academic Medicine,* and appeared in abbreviated form in the February 1992 issue of *The APA Monitor,* the monthly newsletter of the American Psychological Association. We mailed a short note with the announcement to the deans of 126 allopathic and 15 osteopathic medical schools in the United States and 16 medical schools in Canada to alert their faculty and medical education researchers. We also wrote to a selected group of medical education researchers in the United States, Canada, and Great Britain to remind them of the announcement and encourage them to submit proposals.

To eliminate the potential for personal bias in evaluating the anticipated manuscript submissions, seven researchers in medical education who have records of academic publication were invited to serve as special reviewers. We developed a rating form* for the reviewers' use. It required them to rate independently on a seven-point Likert-type scale each of 14 aspects of each manuscript. Sufficient space for comments was also provided. This evaluation format yielded comparable ratings that allowed objective selection of papers for the monograph.

---

*The reviewer evaluation form was adapted from a similar form developed by Dr. Rick Crandall, the Editor of the *Journal of Social Behavior and Personality*.

The seven reviewers each agreed to review a maximum of six manuscripts and to return their evaluations within six weeks. Each reviewer was given the option to review either empirical or theoretical papers or both. The rating forms and instructions for their use were sent to the reviewers with the submitted manuscripts. The names of the papers' authors and their institutional affiliations were erased from the manuscripts for blind review. Each paper was reviewed by at least two reviewers.

Many investigators submitted proposals, and those whose ideas were relevant to the theme were invited to pursue their plans. To reduce methodologic variation and for other reasons described in the introductory article ("A Case of Mistaken Identity"), we sent a proposed research methodology to those investigators whose medical schools had longitudinal databases on their students and graduates and who were interested in contributing empirical papers. Similarity of the hypotheses tested and the methods used to test them would allow combining the mass of data from different databases for meta-analysis (see Epilogue). We encouraged the investigators to use their own data to test three specific hypotheses in addition to their intended hypotheses:

1. Objective measures of knowledge attainment in medical school and those one year after graduation from medical school are highly correlated.
2. Low and high academic standings in medical school are directly and significantly associated with corresponding standings in clinical competence ratings in residency.
3. Such associations are stronger for conceptually similar than for dissimilar measures.

In all, 20 completed manuscripts were received, and half of them were considered for inclusion and accepted after recommended revisions. Because the solicitation procedures had been aimed at experts in the field, the papers not selected were rejected mainly because their contents were not directly relevant to the theme of the monograph, rather than on the basis of inferior quality. The final decision on acceptability was based on the reviewers' evaluations, assessments by the editors and reviewers at *Academic Medicine,* and our recommendations.

Our original plan was to include four sections on internal and external evaluations of medical students, evaluations of residents, evaluations of physicians in practice, and finally, the connections among various measures throughout the medical education continuum. We abandoned that plan because we did not receive enough acceptable articles to include all of the sections. After examining the contents of the accepted articles, we decided to group them into nonempirical and empirical sections.

Subsequent to the publication of the monograph as a supplement to *Academic Medicine*, Springer Publishing Company agreed to reprint it as an independent book for distribution to a wider national and international audience. This present volume is a slightly revised and somewhat expanded edition of the original monograph. It has been expanded by including a foreword by Dr. George E. Miller, a well-known authority in medical education, and by including a commentary section as a closing chapter.

HIGHLIGHTS OF THE CONTENTS

This volume begins with the foreword by Dr. Miller in which it is suggested that although conventional wisdom indicates that the best predictor of future performance is past performance, social, economic and cultural realities should also be considered influential factors in health care. In the foreword to the original edition, Dr. Kassebaum suggests that for the purpose of accreditation, as well as for political and social accountability, medical schools must show that they systematically evaluate their educational outcomes.

Because of her extensive involvement in medical education research and her particular interest in our theme, Christine McGuire was invited to prepare an essay drawn from her experience. Her article addresses important issues in assessment and recommends areas for future research. In the next article, we summarize pertinent information from the literature and describe limitations in empirical findings that prevent the relationships reported from attaining their maximum values.

Nonempirical perspectives on implications of physician evaluation for undergraduate and graduate medical education are described in two articles in Part II. Nash, Markson, Howell, and Hildreth describe three nontraditional methods of physician assessment that are being implemented in the United States. Marshall reports an Australian experience in evaluating the cognitive, affective, and psychomotor performances of family physicians. The last article in this section is an opinion piece by Vogel who discusses the relevance to medical practice of apparently "irrelevant" facts learned in medical school.

Part III contains reports of studies in which the connections between performances before and after graduation from medical school were measured empirically.

In the study reported in the first article of this section, Markert investigated the three hypotheses described above and confirmed all three. Two research questions in the Arnold and Willoughby study addressed the same hypotheses, and their findings support the hypotheses. Vu, Distlehorst, Verhulst, and Colliver report the sensitivity and specificity of the relationships and conclude that scores on examinations in medical school are significantly associated with ratings of clinical competence at the end of the first residency year. The results of the study by Fincher, Lewis, and Kuske also support the hypothesis of significant connections between performances in medical school and ratings of clinical competence in residency.

Case and Swanson found evidence that performances during medical school on standardized examinations of knowledge in the sciences basic to medicine [National Board of Medical Examiners (NBME) Part I] and in the clinical sciences (NBME Part II) were associated with failure rates on certifying examinations, further supporting the relevance of performance in medical school to that in practice. Renschler and Fuchs studied the perceptions of a group of German physicians about the proportions of their knowledge obtained in different phases of medical training. Although these physicians perceived that preclinical and clinical education at university accounted for a median of only about 15% of their knowledge and skills in practice, this small portion of knowledge and skills could have been the foundation of higher-order skills, supporting the proposition of the relevance of knowledge and skills acquired in medical school.

Verhulst and Distlehorst describe the nonresponse bias in a residency follow-up study, an important methodologic limitation that could confound measurement of the full range of competence and reduce the correlations between performance measures in medical school and those in residency.

The article by Taylor and Albo is a reflection on the well-known Utah study that reported no significant association between measures of performance in medical school and physicians' clinical competence. The original study is often cited by medical education researchers, including many authors who have contributed to this monograph. Some of the methodologic and conceptual factors described in our introductory article offer possible reasons for such findings of no association.

In the closing article of this section, we confirm the associations between levels of performance in medical school and clinical competence in residency. We also report our finding that board certification rates were significantly associated with preclinical performances in medical school.

The magnitudes of the associations reported in this monograph are insufficient to prove a large overlap between levels of performance before and after graduation from medical school. We describe in chapter 2 ("A Case of Mistaken Identity") some of the reasons a large overlap has not been consistently reported. Using the analogy of a half-full or a half-empty glass, we continue to be optimistic and view the glass as half full. Indeed, the data reported here suggest that the glass must be more than half-full.

Chapter 16 contains perspectives from international leaders in the profession: Bingxun Liu, M.D. (China), Charles Boelen, M.D. (Switzerland), David M. Macfadyen, M.B.ch.B., F.R.C.P. (Denmark), and Horacio J.A. Rimoldi, M.D., Ph.D. (Argentina) prepared thoughtful commentaries on this volume.

J.S.G.
M.H.
J.B.E.
J.J.V.

PART ONE

Background

Medical education cannot be described or discussed apart from general education.

Abraham Flexner
1866–1959

CHAPTER ONE

Perspectives in Assessment

Christine McGuire

The search for understanding is never disinterested. Success in predicting the course of any phenomenon under study is valued precisely because it furnishes the basis for influencing the phenomenon or, where that is not possible, for mitigating its consequences. This is especially urgent with respect to the psychosocial complexities of medical education as related to clinical practice—hence the seemingly never-ending quest for reliable measures of performance that can be employed to predict the lifelong professional conduct of applicants to medical school and residency training.

Success in this exceedingly important search would expedite selection of the most promising aspirants—those with the greatest potential for completing their medical and specialty education with distinction in the prescribed time, thereby minimizing the social investment required. It would also enable programs to identify persons most likely to choose careers in the geographic and specialty areas of greatest need, thus maximizing the social benefit of the investment.

Decades of research confirm the commonsense observation that much of human behavior is reasonably predictable and that the best indicator of an individual's future conduct in a particular situation is his or her current response to a similar condition; indeed, without such experiential continuity, attempts at social interaction would be attended by intolerable levels of uncertainty.

Nevertheless, our search for predictors of professional performance has met with only very limited success. In the myriad studies repeatedly undertaken by the Association of American Medical Colleges (AAMC), the National Board of Medical Examiners (NBME), several specialty societies, and numerous undergraduate institutions, no strong relationship has been consistently demonstrated between performances at different levels of training, or between in-training performance and clinical practice. Specifically, none of these studies has identified any combination of useful predictors of "success" in practice, however "success" at that level is defined. With the notable exception of the investigation by Gonnella and Hojat,[45] no combination of variables representing performance at the undergraduate level has been found in any study to explain more than about 5% of the variance at the residency level (and that only for the first year of graduate training).

The exception is notable not only for the highly unusual finding that, depending on the specialty, up to 25% of the variance on selected performance variables in the first year of residency could be explained by a combination of third- and fourth-year grades and scores on NBME Part II; the study is also interesting for its methodology, which may help to account for the results. Specifically, (1) no attempt was made to predict overall performance; and (2) data were separately analyzed for each of the three specialties studied.

In general, the strongest relationship so far documented in the continuum of medical education has been observed in the correlations between various combinations of criteria for admission and selection [Medical College Admission Test (MCAT) score and premed grade-point average (GPA)] and class rank in medical school, but even at this level the predictor variables rarely account for more than one-third of the variance in grades on basic science courses, and only 5% to 10% of the variance in clerkship assessments. Although they regularly achieve statistical significance, these reported relationships are too weak to be of much practical value in guiding selection decisions once the relatively few clearly unsuitable candidates have been eliminated from consideration.

PROBLEMS IN PREDICTION

There are at least four general explanations for what, given the social importance of the issue, can only be viewed as disappointing results: (1) limitations imposed by restriction of range; (2) the choice of predictor and criterion variables and their operational definitions; (3) the instrumentation employed in measuring the variables selected; and (4) the role of intervening experience and situational constraints in altering performance differentially.

Restriction of Range

It has been noted repeatedly that, despite increasing diversity in race, gender, and socioeconomic status, medical school applicants are pretty homogeneous with respect to their aptitudes (what the Educational Testing Service increasingly defines as "trained abilities") for the study and practice of medicine. It is probably safe to assume that, with enough time and a reasonably supportive environment and barring any unforeseen catastrophe, nearly everyone who applies is capable of completing medical training. Under these circumstances, and given the exceedingly limited range in the abilities of those who are actually admitted, it is unreasonable to expect high correlations between measures of performance at different times, even on the same tasks. This suggests that we will need to consider methodologies other than correlational and regression analysis in our studies of relationships in performances over time at different levels of medical training and practice.

Selection and Definition of Criteria

While there may be a broad consensus about the general nature of the relevant variables that define success at various points in the medical education continuum, attempts to operationalize them usually reveal unacceptable vagueness, serious limitations in our understanding, and/or basic differences in the meanings we assign. For example, successful completion of medical school in a normal four-year period is widely accepted as an appropriate criterion (with grades in the basic sciences as an intervening variable) against which to measure the utilities of various predictors (e.g., premedical GPA and MCAT score). Attending staff physicians' ratings of residents, particularly in the first postgraduate year, are generally regarded as reasonable criteria against which to measure the validities of such selector variables as NBME examination scores and class rank in medical school.

However, success in clinical practice has been less amenable to easy definition either conceptually or logistically. Although it is generally agreed that the ultimate measure of clinical performance is the quality of care rendered, as indicated by the health status of the population served, other factors (e.g., cost-benefit) must be considered. Even if patient outcome could be accurately determined, differences in the natures of the populations served by individual physicians would vitiate any attempt to compare their performances on such a variable, as witness the criticisms of analogous efforts by the Health Care Financing Administration (HCFA) to rank hospitals on the basis of their mortality rates.

So the question arises as to the availability of other more accessible indicators of quality of care. Most often proposed are so-called "process" criteria, that is, compliance with generally agreed protocols for the work-up and management of patients who present with specified complaints and diagnostic problems. Unfortunately, this approach has also proved to be of limited value in individual assessment, for three reasons: (1) the nature and variety of the problems on which performance must be sampled in order to be able to generalize to the relevant universe of practice; (2) the very large number of cases (estimated to range upward to ten or more observations in a single setting) required to obtain a stable measure of the quality of an individual's decisions with respect to even one diagnostic category; and (3) the inadequate documentation of the relationship between specified diagnostic and/or therapeutic procedures and patient outcomes.

Problems in Instrumentation

No matter how it is defined, professional success at any level is a function of a complex combination of cognitive abilities, prior experience, sensorimotor and interpersonal skills, and various motivational and affective attitudes. Hence, psychometricians have responded to the challenge of providing more valid and reliable evaluations of professional competence by developing techniques for assessing these characteristics.[62,63,120,130]

However, instruments to measure performance during training (both graduate and undergraduate) have, for the most part, been limited to tests of cognitive achievement, supplemented in the clinical years with faculty ratings in some programs. Performance in practice has, in the past, been deduced from proxy measures such as participation in continuing education and self-reports of scientific reading and other professional activities, supplemented in some settings by needs assessments based on chart audits of hospital and/or office records. For purposes of relicensure and recertification, these traditional indices have been expanded in some specialties to include conventional tests of information as well as innovative simulations of office and hospital practice. Unfortunately, as employed, each of these types of instruments has serious deficiencies not only as a predictor of future performance, but even as a method of determining current status, as summarized below.

Formal Testing Programs

First, all tests of any consequence are inherently measures of *maximum,* not *habitual,* performance. Second, only a very few, primarily those developed with professional assistance for national application, meet even minimally acceptable psychometric standards of validity, reliability, and objectivity.

Improvement in Traditional Test Formats

Beginning in the early 1950s the NBME, under the foresighted direction of Dr. John P. Hubbard, led the movement away from the then-prevalent open-ended oral and essay examinations to more objective, reliable and heuristically adequate multiple-choice formats. This dedicated effort contributed significantly to improvements not only in the purely technical characteristics of national licensure and certification examinations but also in the quality of faculty-developed tests produced at the local level.

Further, in response to mounting criticism that, despite their apparent sophistication, these tests required candidates to demonstrate only the ability to recall fragments of isolated information rapidly and under stress—a necessary but woefully insufficient precondition of complex practice—the NBME commissioned a landmark study, the "Critical Performance Requirements of Interns and Residents," which provided a rationale for redesigning its Part III examination. On the basis of this important research, the NBME initiated, in the early 1960s, cautious experimentation with new test formats such as the Film Test*, designed to measure interpretive skills, and the Programmed Test+, used to sample decisions in patient management. Unfortunately, due both to numerous logistical difficulties and to what at times seemed to be a compulsive obsession with extraordinarily narrow issues of reliability, this promising development was gradually vitiated to the point of virtual abandonment in examinations prepared under the auspices of NBME.

---

*The Film Test consisted of a set of exercises, each based on a brief movie clip portraying portions of the physical examination of a patient, followed by a series of multiple choice questions requiring the student to interpret the findings displayed.

+The Programmed Test consisted of a set of exercises, each introduced by a brief statement of a patient complaint and/or related findings, followed by a series of questions about next steps in the work-up or management of the patient. The student recorded the answer to each question in a manner that revealed the patient's response to the chosen intervention, data that were potentially useful for subsequent decisions.

Early Innovation

Concern about the type of competence demanded of examinees continued to surface, and the mid-1960s witnessed a flowering of radically new approaches to instrument design, especially stimulated by research and development at the University of Illinois College of Medicine and several collaborating specialty boards, most notably the American Board of Orthopedic Surgery, the Family Physicians of Canada, and the Committee on Certification in Child Psychiatry of the American Board of Psychiatry and Neurology.

These organizations pioneered a variety of types of simulations in written, oral, and computer formats. Following standard principles of simulation, each exercise was designed so as to present the test stimulus as realistically as feasible, to allow the examinee maximum flexibility in responding, and to alter the resulting situation so as to reflect each individual's choice of action. Thus, in tests of interpretive skill the candidate was presented with physiologic data in the form of laboratory reports; visual data in the form of X-rays, EKG tracings, photographs of lesions, and movies and videotape films of physical examinations; and auditory input in the form of pulmonary, cardiac, abdominal, and other sounds played through individual stethophones. Analogously, structured oral examinations designed to assess communication skills required the candidate, for example, to elicit the history from a simulated patient (i.e., the examiner or a trained layman playing the role of a patient) or to explain something to a "patient" and gain his or her cooperation in a plan of management. Similarly, clinical judgment was tested by written, oral, or computer exercises constructed in the form of branching problems in patient management (PMPs) in which the condition of the simulated patient changed and the problem evolved differently, in accord with the examinee's decisions at each stage in the work-up and management.

Although these promising efforts evoked considerable interest world-wide, admiration for the system did not lead to its widespread emulation. While various elements were adapted elsewhere, there was no wholesale adoption anywhere, probably as a consequence of the investment of examiners' time and ongoing research required to produce high-quality simulations.

Understandably, initial enthusiasms for this new and seemingly more appropriate instrumentation soon gave way to discouragement with the realization that it offered no readily available panacea. Perhaps the most important legacies of this period of innovation are: (1) the continuing sensitivity it created with regard to issues concerning "what it is that a particular test really measures"; (2) visceral recognition that competence is not a simple aggregate of homogeneous performances, but is multidimensional; (3) willingness to admit that such cherished concepts as a "generalized problem-solving skill" may be merely convenient but misleading constructs; and (4) an ongoing concern with the impact of tests on student learning and the effects of different types of examinations on student and candidate priorities and methods of study.

Recent Developments

Current trends require new allegiances. As "performance testing"* is adopted as the new mantra of the cognoscenti, OSCE (objective structured clinical examination), SP (standardized patient), and SCE (simulated clinical encounter) have become the salient acronyms of the 1980s and 1990s, replacing the PMP (patient management problem) so popular in the 1960s and 1970s.

The OSCE, as initially conceived and described by Ronald Harden and his associates at the Centre for Medical Education, Dundee, Scotland, was designed to assess very specific skills (e.g., interpreting an X-ray, palpating the abdomen, or eliciting the presenting complaint from a patient). A total examination consisting of 10 to 20 "stations," at each of which students were allowed a specified time (3–5 minutes) to perform a single, concrete, standardized task, could be objectively administered to very large classes (up to 1200–1500 students in some third-world countries).

More recently this concept has been expanded to include the 20- to 50-minute SCE** in which the examinee is instructed to perform the complete initial work-up of a real or simulated "patient," who is programmed to present all examinees with a standard stimulus representing exactly the same clinical problem. At about the same time that Paula

---

* The term "performance test," though near to achieving recognition as an indispensable part of our technical vocabulary, appears to reflect a naive disregard for plain English: Any response to any test including the much maligned "blacken the answer space corresponding to" is a "performance." To ignore this fact is to risk misinterpreting the results; except perhaps in the case of the National Spelling Bee and the Olympic tryouts, no one is really interested in an individual's test performance per se; rather we are concerned about the conclusions we can draw, and the predictions we can make, on the basis of that "performance."

**The controversy among proponents of this method as to whether the "patient" in question is a "programmed patient," a "standardized patient," or a "simulated patient" appears to be approaching resolution with a near consensus to refer to the test stimulus as a "standardized patient" (SP), and the test situation as a "simulated clinical encounter" (SCE).

Stillman, under the auspices of the American Board of Internal Medicine, was pioneering its experimental use with residents in varied sites, the SCE was being introduced as a certification mechanism at the undergraduate level by Howard Barrows, Reed Williams, and their associates at the Southern Illinois University School of Medicine; currently the potential benefits and feasibility problems of using the SCE in national testing programs is being investigated in a comprehensive study sponsored by the NBME and the Educational Council for Foreign Medical Graduates. In all these manifestations the technique has received detailed scrutiny, and there is now an extensive literature available about it.

Both the OSCE and the SCE have the advantage of presenting the examinee with a standard series of realistic stimuli and of making it feasible to test large numbers of candidates in an objective manner on standardized material. However, like other instruments, each is limited in the types of tasks, problems, or skills that can be sampled in the chosen format. Furthermore, total reliance on the SCE modality, with its lengthier stations, seriously limits the number as well as the variety of problem situations that can be presented within the time allotted. Finally, as with all other instruments, the relevant question is: What can we conclude about an individual's competence on the basis of his or her responses to a particular "performance test?" The same questions as to generalizability, validity, and feasibility that have haunted more conventional testing must also be answered about these newer instruments, none of which has been in large-scale use long enough to assess its contribution to accurate prediction of performance in practice.

Rating Scales

As now employed to evaluate student clerks and housestaff, these instruments range from the global ratings (outstanding, satisfactory, unsatisfactory) used in some institutions; through those that merely list several more or less independent factors (e.g., "use of the laboratory," "clinical judgment," "relations with patients," "willingness to assume responsibility") and those that provide detailed definitions of the several factors and/or descriptions of what constitutes outstanding, acceptable, and unsatisfactory behavior with respect to each; to those that approach the specificity of a check list. The more detailed and descriptive reports are helpful in providing students with feedback useful in improving their skills; however, such instruments are of only limited value in ranking their current, or predicting their future, performances.

First, the lack of consensus among raters on the meanings of criteria and the definitions of standards makes all comparisons dubious. These problems are exacerbated by the well-known "halo effect": the tendency to rate an individual at about the same level on all factors no matter how carefully these have been defined, or how variable the individual's performance. Other considerations include the oft-documented tendency to avoid extremes in rating and especially to eschew negative judgments in our increasingly litigious climate, which further limits the utility of these instruments. As commonly employed, ratings appear to add little to the accuracy of student and/or practitioner assessments. Efforts to create better appraisal devices of this type and to train faculty and staff to use them more reliably have, to date, met with only limited success at best.

Chart Audit

Informal assessment by peers, especially of practitioners working in hospital and group-practice settings, is not new to the medical profession. Traditionally, hospitals have established regular bodies (such as the tissue committee, the abortion committee, the drug committee, and the like) and have given each responsibility for reviewing some aspect of hospital care and for reporting to hospital administrators any significant departures from "accepted practice." The demands for more systematic peer assessment came initially from within the profession. As early as 1960, the Board of Trustees of the American Medical Association (AMA) adopted the official position that hospital medical staffs are responsible for evaluating "the quality of medical care on the basis of documented evidence to support diagnoses, treatment and justified utilization of hospital facilities."

During the 1960s it became increasingly common for hospital staffs, specialty societies, and others to require evidence of participation in continuing education as a condition for retention of membership, and regular involvement in such programs was mandated even by some certification and licensure authorities. These requirements led, in turn, to rapid expansion in the number of recognized courses of continuing medical education, accompanied by a demand from numerous authorities in the field for more relevant and effective programs. In response, various modes of record audit were developed to identify deficiencies in patient care that could be targeted in highly individualized educational offerings.

In 1970, the AMA proposed that local "peer review organizations" of physicians be established to monitor the quality of care and the use of medical services. In the same year, the Joint Commission on Accreditation of Hospitals added a requirement that, as a condition of accreditation, a hospital must have an ongoing medical audit to examine the outcomes as well as the process of care. In 1970, the National Center for Health Services Research and Development, a division of what was then known as the Department of Health, Education and Welfare, anticipating that the Congress might well legislate some form of mandatory review of the quality of medical care in federal programs, initiated and funded the Experimental Medical Care Review Organizations (EMCROs). And, in 1972, Congress did enact legislation requiring the establishment of "professional standards review organizations"—the memorable PSROs—"to monitor the appropriateness of health services financed by the federal government."

Encouraged and supported by the federal government, many quality-of-care studies were undertaken by EMCROs and PSROs across the country. These studies confirmed not only that the medical audit is subject to the above-cited generic difficulties inherent in using "quality of care" as a criterion of performance but also that the results are subject to varied interpretations depending on the specific nature of the investigative technique. For example, it was regularly found that many more physicians were judged to be meeting acceptable standards when implicit (i.e., global) outcome criteria were employed than when explicit process criteria were used, and in the latter case, far fewer physicians were deemed satisfactory when criteria were based on optimal care than when standards were empirically derived from "generally accepted practice." Furthermore, results also differed significantly when the performance index (a numerical indicator of level of compliance with accepted standards) was calculated positively in terms of percentage of indicated actions taken by a physician in a given case from when it was calculated negatively as the number of major departures from the agreed protocol in that case.

Despite difficulties of interpretation, adaptations of the medical audit have been recommended by some specialty societies for purposes of recertification. However, the audit is generally deemed to be more useful in identifying extreme individual deficiencies and widespread deviations amenable to educational or other regulatory interventions. Because of the variable interpretations to which it is subject and the large number of cases (and/or judges) required to reach a stable estimate, there is considerable hesitation about using chart audit for purposes of assessing overall *individual* competence and predicting future performance.

Intervening Experience and Situational Constraints

Beginning with reports from the University of Illinois College of Medicine in the early 1960s about student performances on their then-innovative comprehensive examinations, and confirmed subsequently in the research on medical problem solving by investigators at Michigan State University and elsewhere, a myriad of studies[121] have documented the low correlations between the performances of an individual on different clinical problems at a given time, and on the same problem at different times, in different settings, or on different instruments (e.g., a simulated encounter versus a chart audit). Although it is somewhat more characteristic of cognitive than of attitudinal and technical components of professional behavior, this phenomenon has been observed at all levels of education and experience and with all types of instruments: written simulations, so-called "high-fidelity" modalities, computerized problems in patient management, chart audits, and/or checklists documenting the physician's actions in an office or hospital setting.

Investigators have offered various hypotheses regarding this ubiquitous finding. Among the most common are variants of the following: (1) that it is a function of the instruments used to appraise clinical decisions; (2) that it is a consequence of medical school instruction focused on disease entities rather than on the understanding of normal physiologic vs. pathologic processes and the application of appropriate problem-solving strategies; (3) that much of what has been termed clinical problem solving is really pattern matching and requires only recognition of specific sets of information; (4) that the ability to access one such set is not related to an ability to retrieve another or to select those most clinically cogent; (5) that a clinician's recent experience with a particular phenomenon will necessarily influence his or her perception of the next patient's diagnosis; and (6) that environmental pressures, consciously or unconsciously, act to alter medical procedures (e.g., the typical physician generally orders more diagnostic tests in a teaching hospital than in a community hospital, and tends to adapt management not only to the apparent needs of the patient but also to the requirements of the patient's insurer).

Whatever the explanation, one conclusion is inescapable: The validity of any assessment of clinical competence will depend on the nature, number, and variety of problems and the range of settings in which performance is sampled.

IMPLICATIONS

For Research

The foregoing account of some of the difficulties inherent in assessing the competences of medical students and practitioners is not intended as a source of discouragement. Rather, it is offered as an invitation for medical educators to join with psychometricians and other experts in developing and implementing more valid research designs that will provide more important, more useful, and more reliable data for decision makers, including admission committees, residency directors, and mentors at all levels of medical education.

To accomplish this important goal, the following components of our present research protocols are in urgent need of improvement:

1. *Selection and definition of criterion variables.* First, it is necessary to consider what we are really trying to predict in admission decisions, in resident selection, and at the point of licensure and certification: achievement as a student?; capacity to acquire essential knowledge and skills?; habits and attitudes in dealing with patients?; clinical judgment in delivering patient care?; and/or career choice and speciality selection?

   It is not enough merely to name the criterion. Once the variable(s) has (have) been selected, it is necessary to define each in operational terms that describe the ways in which persons who meet the criterion differ from those who do not. What, for example, are the components of clinical judgment, and what do persons with superior clinical judgment *do* that distinguishes them from others?

   There are many useful approaches to this task, ranging from those that rely almost exclusively on empirical techniques (e.g., job and task analyses), through those that integrate empiricism and expert judgment in varying combinations (e.g., the critical-incident technique) to those that depend almost entirely on systematic analysis of expert judgment (e.g., the Delphi technique). All of these approaches can be employed to provide significant help in defining our problem.

2. *Selection and interpretation of predictor variables.* Equal attention needs to be given to decisions about predictor variables. For example, we have learned that decisions about minority applicants are more valid when information about MCAT performances is supplemented with reports about other types of achievement. We also know that, for all applicants, information

about prior performance as a student, as measured by premedical GPA, is very helpful in predicting performance as a student in a similar setting (i.e., basic science lecture courses), but is far less useful in predicting performance as a student in the clinics and is essentially useless in predicting performance as an independent practitioner. Basic research on the correlates of different kinds of performances can contribute substantially to improving our decisions at every level of medical education and, given the changing nature of medical practice, such research will require periodic updating.

3. *Selection and implementation of data collection instruments.* Most readers will probably agree that the data collection instruments now employed (GPA, class rank, scores on tests, attendings' ratings, etc.) do not constitute valid measures of the multidimensional competence required in the practice of medicine (the ultimate criterion variable). This is a relatively easy deficiency to correct and one on which, as reported above, substantial progress has already been made. What is now required, in addition to continuing research on the more promising techniques for measuring relevant performance, is the use of these innovative instruments in our prediction studies.

4. *Choice and implementation of improved research methodology and design.* As reported above, most of our prediction studies have been based on some form of correlation and regression analysis using some combination of measurements taken at one point in time (e.g., MCAT scores and premedical GPA) to predict some other *overall* score (e.g., class rank in medical school) achieved at a later date. In my view this represents a simplistic approach that ill serves our primary purpose. Trying, for example, to force rankings of motivation and of prior knowledge into a single combined arbitrary index of "academic aptitude" or similarly to insist that ratings of surgical skill, ability to communicate with patients, discrimination in use of the laboratory, and other unique attributes be weighted and aggregated into some unidimensional scale labeled "overall competence" will, I believe, continue to frustrate our efforts to provide meaningful information to decision makers who need to function at every level of training and practice. Detailed recommendations for reform cannot be provided in this brief essay; perhaps it is enough to suggest here that we could probably profit from learning how to incorporate systematic qualitative data in some form of pattern analysis that would yield

relevant personal profiles of an individual's varied characteristics and achievements as he or she progresses through the several stages of training and practice.

For Decision Makers

Until the results from the research efforts outlined above become more fully available, decision makers at all levels of medical education and practice need to exercise more caution in making judgments about a student's or a physician's overall competence on the basis of reports about a few of his or her cases and/or his or her responses to limited examinations, especially those that involve excessive overt or covert stress or that require the examinee to perform tasks that have little resemblance to the situations about which generalizations are to be made. In essence, admission committees, residency directors, licensure authorities, and specialty boards can put less reliance on evaluations of applicants that are based on relatively few observations of the very limited aspects of competence on which we now claim to be able to provide reasonably reliable and objective data, and can advantageously supplement such data with a variety of responsible qualitative, in-depth assessments.

CONCLUSION

Given the potential economic, social, and other benefits of more accurate prediction of student and physician performances, more insightful selection of medical students and housestaff, and more effective mentoring of trainees, the efforts recommended above should be given high priority by researchers and decision makers at every level of medical education and practice.

ACKNOWLEDGMENTS

The author expresses appreciation to her husband, Jules H. Masserman, M.D., formerly co-chairman and professor, Psychiatry and Neurology, Northwestern University Medical School, for the many helpful suggestions he made during the preparation of this essay.

CHAPTER TWO

A Case of Mistaken Identity: Signal and Noise in Connecting Performance Assessments Before and After Graduation From Medical School

Joseph S. Gonnella, M.D., Mohammadreza Hojat, Ph.D., James B. Erdmann, Ph.D., and J. Jon Veloski, M.S.

Solid evidence of the connections between what students learn in medical school and the quality of their later performances as physicians in practice has thus far eluded the medical community. It may be argued that if such connections cannot be demonstrated empirically, the legitimacy of what is learned in medical school and the need to expend vast resources to provide medical education should be seriously questioned.

The ultimate purpose of education in any profession is to inculcate the knowledge, skills, competence, and other characteristics required for expected performance of that profession. Logically, in a structured and purposeful professional education such as medicine, there must be continuity from one level of training to another. Thus, more advanced levels of training are assumed to be built upon the foundations laid in previous levels, and all the levels are presumed to be relevant to the target professional behavior. In support of this notion, Young[207] stated more than three decades ago that "the study of medicine is a continuous educational program. The formal education in medical schools serves only as a brief, intensive part of the preparation of the physician."

Medical education has the unique feature of being composed of two components, the basic sciences and the clinical sciences. In a majority of medical schools these components are separated chronologically, under the assumption that the clinical component must be built upon a firm foundation of basic sciences. Ironically, while this connection between basic and clinical sciences in medical school is taken for granted, the relationships of academic attainments in the basic sciences and achievements in the clinical sciences, particularly the associations between grades in the basic sciences and performances in practice, have been questioned. Does the uncertainty about these associations truly reflect a real problem, or is this a case of mistaken identity?

REVIEW OF THE LITERATURE

The presumptive continuum between the knowledge and skills obtained in medical school and competence in providing care has not been consistently supported by empirical studies. The issues has long been debated but has not been settled because research findings are inconsistent. For example, based on a review of 27 articles in which the relationships between college grades and later professional performances were empirically investigated (only seven of the articles concerned medicine), Wingard and Williamson[202] concluded that there was little or no correlation between college grades and professional performance.

Extensive literature review as well as empirical analyses by Price and colleagues, published in several monographs, papers and a book[81,144,145,147,156] suggest, in general, a lack of overlap between measures of academic performances and performances in professional medicine. For example, to investigate the relationships between academic measures and indices of practice performances, Price and colleagues[145] reviewed 61 papers, and Jacobsen and colleagues[81] reviewed 148, both concluding that no consistent relationship exists between the two sets of measures. Extensive correlational and factor-analytic studies by Price and colleagues[144,147] led them to assert that performances in medical school and the clinical competences of physicians are independent and that, therefore, no overlap between them would be expected.

One of the reasons proposed by Price and colleagues[147] for the lack of a relationship between performance measures in preclinical years and physician performances was the independence of the mathematically derived factors of the medical school and practice measures used in their study. One may argue that variables clustering under one factor are not necessarily independent of other variables clustering under another factor. In fact, almost all variables used in factor analyses (e.g., basic science variables and clinical ratings of competence in residency) can be correlated, but some of the variables are more correlated than others. Those variables that have higher intercorrelations cluster together and form a factor. The cluster is regarded as different from another cluster whose variables are themselves interrelated. To present a simpler factor pattern, the orthogonal rotation method is frequently used. This calculation creates mathematically independent factors that simplify either the rows of a factor matrix (quartimax method) or the columns of the matrix (varimax method). The mathematical independency of the factors is indeed an artifact of the rotation method. Other types of rotation (oblique rotation) do not create independent factors. Therefore, factor independency can be caused by the chosen rotational method and may not be inherent in the data.

Various investigations have confirmed relationships between measures of performances in medical school and performances after graduation. For example, Gunzburger and colleagues[60] reported that scores on the National Board of Medical Examiners (NBME) Part II examination and performances in clinical clerkships of medicine and surgery were significantly associated with the levels of competence of residents in the first year of residency training. Kegel-Flom[90] found that supervisors' ratings of residents were best forecasted by faculty ratings of students in the third and fourth years of medical school. Significant correlations were also observed between grades in medical school (in basic as well as clinical sciences) and ratings of residents by residency supervisors and peers.[90]

Gough and colleagues[54] found that grade-point averages in medical school were sufficiently reliable and internally homogeneous to be considered an index that related well to other concurrent performance measures and was moderately predictive of performance during residency and at least the early years of practice.

Last and colleagues[102] among others, found a close association between student achievement and subsequently obtaining posts in teaching hospitals in the United Kingdom. Richardson[157] showed that success on examinations in undergraduate medical education was related to higher qualifications four and a half years after graduation, and Wakeford and Roberts[195] suggested a positive but tenuous relationship between performance on medical school examinations and subsequent career success, based on their findings in the United Kingdom. They measured success as the physicians' possession of higher medical credentials, cited publications, prestigious appointments, and fellowships awarded by the Royal College of Physicians.

Weston and Dubovsky[197] reported that first-year residents who had

had academic problems in medical school were rated slightly lower than average by their residency program directors. Yindra and colleagues[206] found statistically significant relationships between achievement measures in medical school and performance ratings in residency. They observed that residents rated "outstanding" had performed better on the NBME examinations (Parts I and II) than residents rated "below average." Based on their results, Yindra and colleagues[206] suggested that performance measures in medical school be considered in the selection of residents, but they cautioned that using them as a single selection factor or as a method of screening applicants from further consideration is justifiable only when medical school achievement is extremely high or low.[206] Johnson and colleagues[84] showed that excellent medical students are more likely to be superior physicians than are mediocre students. They found that the excellent students in their study were among the top 10% of the residents and were more likely than the others to be assistants to the staff. Monk and Thomas[123] reported associations between class standing in medical school and board certification and academic affiliation after medical school.

The question of the relationships between performance measures in medical school and those after graduation was addressed in two investigations based on the Jefferson Longitudinal Study of Students and Graduates.[45,186] Data related to the topic were also presented in several other studies by researchers at Jefferson.[49,66,148,187,210] Veloski and colleagues[186] found that correlations between measures of performance in medical school and ratings of postgraduate competence were statistically significant but small (range .10 to .37). Gonnella and Hojat[45] and Veloski and colleagues[186] reported significant associations between the academic status of students as high or low scorers in medical school and ratings at the top or bottom of a competence rating scale in residency training, respectively. In addition, Gonnella and Hojat[45] found that the relationships between measures of academic achievement in medical school and measures of postgraduate competence vary among specialties and at different performance levels. For example, the associations between the two sets of measures before and after graduation were stronger for residents in internal medicine and obstetrics-gynecology than for residents in pediatrics. Differences in ranges, variability of performance measures, and variability in evaluation standards among specialties were possible reasons for these findings.

Also, the associations between sets of measures before and after graduation were found to be more stable for those at the high and low ends of the score distributions than for those in the middle. Gonnella and Veloski[49] reported that scores on the NBME Part III examination were a function not only of performance on Part II, taken in medical school, but also of the type of residency program pursued in the first postgraduate year before taking Part III. Herman and colleagues[66] found a significant association between low clinical performance ratings in junior clerkships and ratings of a noncognitive area (professional attitudes) after graduation. Turner and colleagues[184] reported associations between the scores on NBME Part I and Part II and postgraduate ratings of medical knowledge. Based on these associations, they suggested a new passing score for the NBME examinations. Veloski and colleagues[187] reported significant correlations between performance measures in medical school and scores on the NBME Part III examination (the correlations ranged from .24 to .70). Rabinowitz and Hojat[148] found that grades on junior clerkship examinations based on essay and multiple choice questions correlated significantly with NBME Part III scores (the correlations ranged from .32 to .49). In this study, clerkship examination grades were also found to correlate with ratings on areas of postgraduate competence, but these were low magnitude correlations (ranging from .11 to .23).

QUALITATIVE AND QUANTITATIVE VIEWS OF THE ISSUE

The connections between academic attainment in medical school and performance in practice can be discussed from both qualitative and quantitative points of view.

Qualitative View

The purposes of medical care can be defined as advocating and implementing the highest standards for prevention and proposing the best possible diagnosis and employing effective treatment for the individual in need of care. The question that must be answered is: when a physician's understanding of anatomic structure, function, neurobiochemical actions, and other basic and clinical sciences concepts is inadequate, can he or she achieve those goals?

Billings, the founder of *Index Medicus,* reported in 1887 that nine-tenths of medical knowledge (basic or clinical) becomes worthless or of no interest within ten years of its publication, and much of it is so when it first appears (cited by Taylor[175]). This certainly does not imply that knowledge should not be acquired on the ground that it is becoming obsolete constantly. New knowledge is always based on old knowledge, and one must not stop learning the current knowledge because of the probability of its transformation in the near future. Assuming this proposition is accepted, then, at least in theory, a foundation of basic science knowledge is required for better understanding of the mechanisms of disease as well as health.

Quantitative View

Reviews of empirical studies, in general, indicate that when statistically significant correlations between measures of performance in medical school and ratings of competence after graduation have been reported, their magnitudes have not been sufficient to support a strong connection. For example, correlations ranged from .15 to .33 in a study reported by Richards and colleagues[156] from .10 to .37 in a study by Veloski and colleagues,[186] and from .13 to .33 in another study by Veloski and colleagues.[187] Gonnella and Hojat[45] found higher multiple correlations when they studied physicians in the specialties of internal medicine and obstetrics-gynecology (correlations ranged from .30 to .51) and nonsignificant correlations when they studied physicians in pediatrics. Therefore, it seems that when measures of academic performance in medical school are correlated with measures of clinical competence after graduation, the relationships are generally positive but relatively slight.

This pattern of findings has also been observed in professions other than medicine.[202] In the area of industrial and organizational psychology, correlations between scores on aptitude tests and job success fall between the .20s and .30s for a variety of jobs.[42] Based on their validity generalization research, Schmidt and Hunter[167] argue that these correlation coefficients are indeed underestimates of the true validity of the tests.

If it is acceptable that a better understanding of medicine requires a solid foundation of knowledge in the basic sciences, then why has a strong relationship between such knowledge acquired in medical school and the competence of a physician not been demonstrated? The question is of paramount importance. Possible answers will clarify, to some extent, the uncertainty surrounding the relationship.

CONTAMINATING FACTORS, CONCEPTUAL AND METHODOLOGIC ISSUES, AND ENHANCING VARIABLES

The lack of large overlap between measures of attainment in medical school and performances after graduation can be partially explained by examining the contributions of contaminating factors and by studying conceptual and methodologic issues. We discuss the contaminators and the conceptual and methodologic elements that produce "noise." "Noise" is defined here as any factor that interferes with attaining the maximal value of the association between attainment in medical school and performance after graduation. Such "noise" obscures the strength of the "signal," which is defined as the maximal relationship (overlap).

We briefly describe those contaminators related to time interval, educational institutions, and specialty areas. Conceptual and methodologic issues are then outlined. Finally, the contribution of noncognitive factors (personal qualities) in enhancing the predictive validities of performances before, during, and after medical school is considered.

Contaminators

Three contaminators obscure the relationships between measures of attainment in medical school and in practice.

Time Interval

Retention of knowledge is a function of the interval between its acquisition and its retrieval.[71] The hypothesis that performances on particular subtests of a comprehensive examination (NBME Part II) would be a function of the length of time between completion of corresponding clerkship training and the administration of the subtests was confirmed in a study of medical students.[71] The phenomenon of "decay of learning" as a function of time has been attributed to a number of sources, including the time factor[17,93,172] According to Peterson and colleagues,[139] better medical students, on the average, performed at higher levels for a few years after entering practice, but this effect weakened over time (p. 55).

One of the pioneering studies of the associations between performances before and after medical school was reported in 1925 by Bott,[16] who concluded that the criterion of achievement to compare with performance after graduation from medical school should be taken from the later rather than the earlier years of medical education. Gaier[40] also emphasized that measures of the clinical science component of medical education (taken later) were more appropriate than were measures of the basic science component (taken earlier) for predicting postgraduate competence.

In a factor-analytic study, Gough and Hall[53] found that the clinical-performance factor was more important than any other academic attainment in medical education in predicting postgraduate clinical competence. Consistent with these findings, Richards and colleagues[156] reported that the best predictor of intern performance was the grade-point average in the clinical years of medical school; grades in the preclinical years had only a slight relationship to intern performance, and premedical grades had almost no relationship. This pattern of findings could be due either to the time interval between the evaluations or to conceptual similarities of the assessments, discussed later.

Ramsey and colleagues[149] found an inverse correlation between scores from knowledge evaluations and number of years elapsed since certification. The "recency effect" postulates that recall is stronger (assuming no rehearsal) for recently learned information than for information learned earlier.[93,127] Based on this postulation, everything else being equal, it is expected that the early component of medical education will yield a weaker association with performance in residency than the later component, and to a certain degree the associations will diminish as the interval between the assessments becomes longer.

Educational institution

The objectives and contents of the medical school curriculum, the quality of the residency programs, and their interactions contribute to the magnitudes of associations between performance measures in medical school and those in residency and afterward. This explains, in part, the variation in the magnitudes of these associations found for graduates of different institutions. Despite this, Norcini and colleagues[133] reported that knowing more medicine at the time of certification was associated primarily with higher achievement in medical school rather than with the educational experience provided by the residency training program. In a study of Canadian general practitioners, Clute[25] found a significant association between performances in medical school and after graduation in one group of surveyed physicians and a nonsignificant association in another group. Variation in the educational institutions might be one reason, among others, for the contradiction in these results.

Specialization

It has been reported[49] that physicians who pursued broader areas of training (e.g., internal medicine) performed better on the clinical knowledge section of a certifying examination and the patient management section of NBME Part III than did their colleagues in more focused areas (e.g., pathology).[49]

Peterson and colleagues[139] concluded that "upon examination of the physician's academic performance and his hospital training, two facts emerge. First, the better medical student tends to become a better physician. Second, the more training a physician has received in internal medicine, the more likely he is to become a good physician" (p. 143). Gonnella and Hojat[45] observed that the association between performance measures in medical school and residency was stronger for physicians who pursued internal medicine and obstetrics-gynecology than for those who pursued pediatrics. These findings indicate that for particular specialties a stronger connection is expected between knowledge attained in medical school and knowledge used in practice. For other areas of specialization, the connection loses its strength. Possible reasons for this have been discussed elsewhere.[45]

Conceptual Issues

It is evident that the physician's multifaceted role and the multidimensional aspects of patient care are not totally reflected in the academic activities of medical students.[46] The competent practicing physician has not only a foundation of medical knowledge but also a wide assortment of clinical, pedagogical, and managerial skills that are mostly acquired in postgraduate training and practice.

Construct Similarities and Dissimilarities

A physician implicitly plays at least three roles: clinician, educator, and manager.[46,47,50] The knowledge and skills acquired during medical school as well as the physician's attitudes and personal qualities contribute to performance in each of those roles. Obviously, the cognitive knowledge and clinical skills acquired in medical schools have more relevance to the physician's role as a clinician than to his or her role as an educator or manager. This implies that in examining the relationships between performance measures before and after graduation from medical schools, *construct similarities* of the measure produce "signal" and *construct dissimilarities* produce "noise"; hence, one expects stronger or weaker associations, respectively. For example, associations between two measures that are conceptually similar (e.g., knowledge of basic sciences in medical school and knowledge of basic sciences in residency) should be stronger than those between two conceptually dissimilar measures (e.g., knowledge of basic science in medical school and managerial skills in practice).

Empirical data are available in support of this conclusion. For example, Hojat and colleagues[69] used a factor analytic approach to find that knowledge-based examinations in medical school and ratings of competence in medical school loaded on different factors. Based on the rotated factor loadings, it was also observed that competence ratings in residency yielded weaker relationships with the factor of knowledge-based examinations than with global clinical competence ratings in medical school.[69] Zeleznik and colleagues[210] also used the factoranalytic method and reported that performance on examinations in medical school loaded on a factor different from (or orthogonal to) another factor defined by admission measures (undergraduate grade-point averages and levels of recommendation contained in the letters of recommendation); both factors were orthogonal to a third factor describing clinical competence ratings in residency.

Gough and Hall[53] concluded that a factor they called "clinical performance" was more important than any other academic attainment measure in medical school in predicting postgraduate clinical competence. Korman and Stubblefield[95] reported that grades in medical school were inadequate indicators in predicting ratings of residents, but ratings of peers in medical school were related to the competence ratings in residency.

Keck and colleagues[89] reported significant correlations among scores on NBME Part II (clinical knowledge examination) instructors' evaluations in the internal medicine clerkship, and ratings of the clinical competence of physicians. They did not find a significant correlation between scores on NBME Part I (basic science knowledge examination) and ratings of postgraduate competence. Richards and colleagues[156] reported that the best predictor of intern performances was grades in the clinical year (third year) of medical school, and that grades in the preclinical years of medical school had only a slight relationship to intern performances.

Data on numerous performance variables in medical school and after graduation indicate that examination grades load on a factor conceptually different from those loaded on by ratings of clinical performance in medical school and by ratings of clinical competence after graduation.[69] These dissimilarities in constructs, or in factors, are likely to be responsible for the shrinkage of correlations between the two sets (before and after graduation from medical school), that is, the relationships' failure to reach their maximal values. Thus, conceptual dissimilarities create a different type of noise that reduces the strength of the signal.

Methodologic Issues

As we reported elsewhere,[46,47,69] correlations between measures of performances before and after graduation from medical school are also subject to methodologic problems.

Bivariate Normal Distribution

The theory of correlation has close ties with the normal distribution. One aspect of a bivariate normal distribution (when using Pearson correlation) is that the distributions of both the dependent and the independent variables are normal (bell-shaped). However, it has been reported that ratings of clinical performance are characterized by a negatively skewed distribution.[186,204] One reason given for the negative skewness is the "leniency" or "ceiling" effect, which is defined as the tendency to systematically give high ratings to colleagues when using a rating form. Correlations based on skewed distributions cannot attain their maximum values.[23]

Linearity

The Pearson product-moment correlation technique assumes that the means of one variable for separate scores of the other variable fall on a straight line. In other words, the relationship between two variables should be linear. The linearity assumption can be tested by inspecting the scatter diagram of the dependent and independent variables. In one empirical investigation of the linearity assumption (relating medical school performance and rating of postgraduate competence), departure from linearity was not confirmed.[69] However, since a nonlinear (curvilinear) relationship between variables may produce (under the linearity assumption) a correlation that is misleading and close to zero, it is always a good practice to test the linearity assumption, at least by inspecting the scatter diagrams.[43]

Homoscedasticity

Skewed distributions and departure from linearity may also result in a departure from homoscedasticity, which assumes that the variance in one variable is the same at all values of the other variable. In other words, it is assumed that the standard deviation of the dependent variable remains the same, regardless of the specified value of the independent variable.[113] When homoscedasticity is absent, the extent of the relationship cannot be totally captured by the correlational coefficient.[182] Therefore, the results based on correlation analysis will underestimate the extent of relationships between the variables. We observed an absence of homoscedasticity in an empirical study examining relationships between measures before and after graduation from medical school.[69]

Restriction of Range

The correlation coefficient is highly dependent upon the range and variability of measured values in the sample. With everything else being equal, the less the variability or the range of scores in a particular sample, the lower the correlation.[59] Inferences drawn from many of the retrospective studies in medical education are limited by the biasing effects of selection and attrition at every level of medical education and practice. Variation in the performances of medical graduates is limited first by admission criteria, which rely heavily upon prior academic achievement, and then by evaluation mechanisms used in medical school and residency programs that further restrict the range of performance. These selection procedures result in a more homogeneous group, which is reflected in a narrower range of scores and less variation. Although statistical corrections have been suggested for correlations resulting from restricted scores,[69] such corrections are questionable.[39,211]

Multicollinearity

In addition to methodologic issues related to bivariate correlations, another problem arises when using multiple-regression techniques where the predictors are highly intercorrelated. This problem, called multicollinearity,[29] is particularly serious when the correlations between predictors and criteria are substantially lower than intercorrelations among the predictors.[51] Reported data indicate that correlations among performance measures in medical school (predictors) are usually higher than those between medical school and residency performances (criterion measures).[187] In extreme cases of multicollinearity (intercorrelations above .80), it is impossible to invert the correlation matrix, precluding calculation of multiple correlations. The situation in which correlations among predictors are extremely high and correlations between predictors and criteria are relatively low creates unstable estimates with high standard errors[38] and should be carefully considered when prediction models are being established.

Different Assessment Methods

Campbell and Fiske[22] described a multitrait-multimethod matrix in which it was observed that correlation between the same attributes was much lower when measured by different methods than when measured by similar methods. They also noticed that different attributes measured by similar methods correlated because of the common method variance. Academic attainments of medical students, particularly in the sciences basic to medicine, have been assessed largely by performances on written examinations, mostly in the multiple-choice format. A similar method is also frequently used to evaluate clinical science knowledge. Ratings of clinical competence have been made in medical school by using observations of skills in controlled clinical situations.

Diverse methods such as objective examinations, ratings, peer review, computer-based examinations, and tests based on simulated or standardized patients have been used to assess physicians' performances. Using the argument presented by Campbell and Fiske,[22] other things being equal, one expects to obtain the highest correlations between performance measures before and after graduation from medical school when the same attribute is evaluated using a similar method of assessment (monotrait-monomethod). In fact, such correlations could be considered as estimates of the reliability of either the trait or the measuring instrument. On the other hand, the lowest correlations, or no relationships, are expected when different attributes are measured using different methods of assessment (heterotrait-heteromethod). The magnitudes of correlations in other situations (monotrait-heteromethod, heterotrait-monomethod) fall between those two ends. This implies that because of the similarity of the assessment methods, knowledge in medical school assessed by objective examinations should correlate better with knowledge assessed by objective examinations taken in residency than with ratings of knowledge in residency or practice.

Published data support this proposition. Calhoun and colleagues[20] found that performances on NBME Part III, taken in residency, had a modest relationship with faculty evaluations of clinical problem solving during medical school, and they reported stronger relationship when NBME Part III scores and the scores on NBME Parts I and II were compared. A similar pattern was found in a large sample study by Veloski, Hojat, and Gonnella.[187] They reported a correlation of .60 when correlating objective examination grades in the third year of medical school with scores on NBME Part III, an objective examination of clinical knowledge and patient management usually taken at the end of the first residency year.[187] The correlation between ratings of clinical competence in the third year and scores on the objective examination of clinical knowledge and patient management in residency (NBME Part III) was .24.[187] This is consistent with expectations with regard to similar and dissimilar methods of assessment.

Nonrepresentativeness as a Result Voluntary Participation

The most sensitive studies of the relationships between medical education and ratings of professional competence are those that allow data to be collected prospectively for the purpose of comparing the performances of students with their later performances as residents and practitioners. In two studies, medical school graduates who had given written permission for the collection of postgraduate data were compared with graduates who had not done so, and it was found that the former group included more high achievers in medical school.[13,69] It was also discovered that permission to collect data after graduation was associated not only with higher performance in medical school[13,69] but also with demographic characteristics such as gender. Women were significantly less likely than men to give such permission.[13] These findings raise questions about the representatives of those who voluntarily participated in the study. They also explain, in part, the ceiling effects (negatively skewed distributions) observed in the postgraduate competence ratings mentioned earlier.

Psychometric Characteristics of Measures of Attainment During Medical School

Other methodologic issues are related to the psychometric properties of the measures being correlated. In this regard, the validity and reliability of the measures are of particular concern. A majority of studies of relationships between measures of performance in medical school and clinical competence do not report supporting evidence of established measurement characteristics for the scores or ratings used (particularly those of clinical competence). It is obvious that invalid or unreliable measures are contaminated by factors that affect the magnitudes of their relationships, creating noise rather than signal.

Measurement Characteristics of Ratings of Postgraduate Competence

Ratings are subjective assessments made on an established scale. They are considered to be rough appraisals of behavior, and it has been argued that they tend to be unreliable, biased, and contaminated.[128] A well-known error in rating is the "halo-effect," that is, the rater's tendency to be influenced by a single favorable or unfavorable trait. Another frequent error is the leniency effect, defined as the reluctance of raters to assign unfavorable ratings. Both the halo effect and leniency errors make ratings less discriminating and distort the magnitudes of correlations when rating scales are used. Despite the limitations inherent in most rating forms, several studies support their construct validity.[45,66,68,92,186]

There is no overall "cure" for all of these methodologic ills. Indeed, some of these difficulties are insurmountable (e.g., restriction of range as a result of selection and attrition is inevitable unless we let all applicants enter and graduate from medical school).

Despite these limitations, there are ways to reduce the methodologic (and conceptual) noise to better elucidate the relationships between the variables. Thus, one solution to the problem of the restrictive statistical assumptions is to employ statistical methods that are less sensitive to the limitations imposed by the skewed distribution of ratings. For example, "distribution-free" statistics (nonparametric statistical methods), although admittedly less powerful, can eliminate some of the methodologic noise, increasing the signal-to-noise ratio.

Also, grouping together all evaluations of diverse knowledge (e.g., basic and clinical sciences) or clinical skills (e.g., data gathering and interpersonal) tends to reduce the specificity aspect of the validity of such composite measures. One solution to this conceptual problem would be to employ factor-analytic techniques to reduce the vast number of performance variables to a few homogeneously meaningful dimensions that can make sense not only statistically but also conceptually. Admittedly, redefinition of the components of a composite measure (by employing a factor-analytic procedure) or the use of less restrictive data analysis (such as a distribution-free statistical method) will not resolve other problems, such as those imposed by the psychometric characteristics of the measurements (e.g., validity and reliability). The standardized measuring instruments and objective examinations used to evaluate knowledge before or after medical school, though limited in the scope of evaluation and validity, will not present serious reliability problems. It is well-known intrinsic deficiencies of rating scales that contribute to the validity and reliability weaknesses of such measures and ultimately confound the signal.

Enhancing Variables

Empirical research in medical education has placed great emphasis on the cognitive dimension of performance (basic and clinical sciences), while the noncognitive (psychosocial) dimension of the personal qualities related to competence and care has been sorely ignored.

Data on the contributions of noncognitive factors to medical school students' and physicians' performances reported by Hojat and colleagues suggest that they are significant.[70,73,209] Including personal qualities enhanced the relationships between performance measures in medical school and in practice.[70,73,209] Keck and colleagues'[89] inclusion of personality measures in their prediction model significantly increased the amount of variance of postgraduate ratings that was explained by the predictors. This phenomenon was also noticed when personality measures were added to the admission measures in predicting performances in the first and second years of medical school and on NBME Part I.[73] Kegel-Flom[90] found that peer ratings of residents were best predicted by a combination of personal inventory measures.

Hunt and colleagues[76] compared the performances of residents who had had academic difficulties in medical school (considered for dismissal or probation) with those of their counterparts without such difficulties. The residents who had had academic difficulties generally received lower ratings than did the other residents on items measuring knowledge and skills, but the observed differences were not statistically significant except on one item dealing with the quality of interaction with patients. The residents who had had academic difficulties were rated significantly lower than their counterparts on this item.

Although conventional measures of undergraduate academic abilities have been shown to relate significantly to examination grades in the basic science component of medical education (usually the first two years in medical school), they do not correlate as well with evaluations of the clinical science component (usually the last two years in medical school) or ratings of performance after graduation.[69]

Empirical findings suggest that measures of postgraduate competence include both cognitive and noncognitive dimensions.[72] Further, a noncognitive factor such as interpersonal relationships is a better predictor of further residency offers than is a cognitive factor.[68] Kupfer and colleagues[100] reported that measurements of academic achievement and personality style represent a better approach to predicting which medical students will make better clinicians. Render and Jackson[151] reported similar findings for students in veterinary school. Gough and Hall,[52] in a study of predictors of who would and who would not graduate from medical school, found that personality measures and academic ability together were the best predictors. Weston and Dubovsky[197] reported that medical students who had emotional problems in medical school were rated lowest on the areas of postgraduate competence. Williams[198] reported an association between personality measures and vocational choice in medical students, and Murden and colleagues[126] suggested that emphasizing the personal characteristics of medical school applicants can increase the prediction of success in the clinical years.

Reinhardt and Gray[150] and Yufit, Pollack, and Waserman[208] reported that personality is a salient factor in the socialization of medical students and physicians that should receive more attention. Levinson[107] suggested that both personality and situational factors should be studied in medical education. Linn and Zeppa[108] found that externality in locus of control and lower self-esteem affect medical students' perceptions of stress, and Huebner, Roger, and Moore[75] spoke of dysfunctional stress and its disturbing effects on medical students' performances.

These empirical findings strongly suggest that the role of personal qualities in shaping clinical competence should not be treated with benign neglect in medical education research. The argument should be revitalized by further defining and studying personal qualities pertinent to medicine. Psychometrically sound instruments should either be developed or be adapted to measure objectively those factors that can be related conceptually and empirically to the construct of a physician's clinical competence.

Maximizing the Signal, Minimizing the Noise

The strength of the association between performances before and after graduation from medical school can be improved by reducing the error variance caused by the confounding factors we have described. The ratio of signal to noise will be maximized when the noise is minimized.

It seems almost impossible to extricate empirically the tangled web of the extraneous elements that obscure the area of overlap between performances before and after graduation. An elegant experimental design is necessary to enhance common variations caused by the independent (performance during medical school) and dependent (performance after medical school) variables and to control for the confounding variables (e.g., variations due to time interval, format similarity, conceptual relevance, training institutions, and methodologic and range restrictions). Implementing such a design is neither practical nor ethical. Such a design would require, for example, that medical schools graduate those students who fail so that the range of performances of graduates would not be restricted statistically. The predicament does not mean that we are hopeless or helpless in determining the extents of the relationships among the measures. If we cannot determine the maximum or optimal variations in the relationships, we can still show improvements by controlling for one, or two, or a few sources of error variance at a time; or, where control of such error variance is impossible, we can at least be aware of it. Awareness can at least prevent the drawing of erroneous conclusions, given known limitations.

CONCLUSION

It is clear from the foregoing considerations that we have not been careful enough in our studies of the connection between performances before and after graduation from medical school. We have not been sufficiently scrupulous with our operational definitions of predictor and criterion variables. Consequently, we have not identified the best instruments for collecting the data or the best methods for analyzing them.

In short, researchers have not really been studying the problem they assumed they were studying. It is really a case of mistaken identity, a failure to identify the problems properly, including the contaminating as well as enhancing factors and several conceptual and methodologic issues. The signal is there but it may be obscured by the background noise. Future research will need to take account of the issues raised in this review in order to identify accurately the magnitudes of the connections among performance assessments at the various stages of medical education.

PART TWO

Nonempirical Perspectives

Appearances to the mind are of four kinds:
Things either are what they appear to be; or they neither are, nor appear to be; or they are, and do not appear to be; or they are not, yet appear to be.
Rightly to aim in all these cases is the wise man's task.

Epictetus
Greek philosopher of the first century A.D.

CHAPTER THREE

Evaluating the Competence of Physicians in Practice: From Peer Review to Performance Assessment

David B. Nash, M.D, M.B.A.,
Leona E. Markson, Sc.D., Susan Howell, M.S.S.,
and Eugene A. Hildreth, M.D., M.A.C.P.

Physicians critique decisions made by colleagues at all levels of training in the continuum from medical school through residency to practice. This process of review by one's peers has come under increasing scrutiny in an era marked by skyrocketing health care costs and calls for major system reforms. Traditional peer review may soon give way to actually assessing physician performance.

This evolutionary process to replace peer review may meet strong resistance in many teaching hospitals, where the routine of the late morning concludes with attending rounds. By the time the corporate world takes its mid-morning coffee break, house officers and medical students have seen all of their hospitalized patients, analyzed dozens of laboratory findings, reviewed several diagnostic tests, and perhaps have even spoken with one or two subspecialty consultants. Now, with the teaching attending physician present, the team members will review their findings again, discuss the intricacies of the differential diagnosis, and arrive at a patient care plan for the next 24 hours. This rich intellectual exercise with layers of review and re-review has been the cornerstone of in-hospital learning for trainees and educators alike.[97]

BACKGROUND

Despite nearly five decades of experience with this pedagogic model, some recent evidence about physicians' collective performance is very disheartening. Trainees make mistakes; indeed, all physicians would acknowledge this as inevitable, yet in one study only 54% of house officers ever discussed their mistakes with the attending physicians and only 24% told the patients or families.[205] Trainees self-report[185] high levels of interest in learning the rudiments of risk management, professional liability, and quality assurance, but little formal exposure to these concepts occurs during residency.[3]

Trainees are not alone. In a broad review of tens of thousands of inpatient charts across more than 50 hospitals, Brennan and colleagues[18] found that there "is a substantial amount of injury to patients from medical management, and many injuries are the result of substandard care." Subsequent studies by the same team[105] suggest that many adverse patient events are potentially preventable now through several mechanisms, including a heavy emphasis on "systems analysis" and education coupled with practice guidelines.

Outside the walls of major academic medical centers and community teaching hospitals lies the largely closed realm of office-based practice. Little formal work, on a national scale, has evaluated the quality of medical care and adverse events in the outpatient setting.

Peer assessment, as illustrated in the aforementioned scenarios, is the cornerstone of assuring and evaluating the quality of medical care across practice settings once physicians leave their training programs and start practice. Yet, the process and tools of peer review have recently fallen under attack. Goldman[44] has urged a "global re-examination" of the peer-review process after finding that physician agreement regarding quality of care is only slightly better than the level expected by chance. In contrast, the academic training model is based on a hierarchical evaluation system and less on peer review. The attending physicians review one another's performances *and* the work of the house officers, who in turn supervise the medical students.

Recently, the peer review process mandated by federal law and conducted through peer review organizations (PROs) has been found wanting because of a marked variability in procedure-specific review criteria and the fact that the criteria differ significantly from identified practice guidelines.[91] In addition, when compared with an independent panel of credible judges on the quality of care, the initial screening process of a PRO failed to detect and refer for PRO physician review two of three records that this one study judged substandard.[163]

As suggested by Langsley, "A nation that spends 12 % of its gross national product on health care demands that the quality of such services be examined and that payment be denied for unneeded or incompetent care by a physician. The era of irrevocable licensure and lifetime certification has given way to the call for periodic specialty recertification and medical relicensure on the basis of performance assessment."[101] In this paper, we illustrate how such a national system for performance assessment is evolving by examining three distinct programs that assess performance in the individual physician's office, in the hospital setting, and collectively at the state level. The relationships between these evaluation systems for practicing physicians are discussed in terms of opportunities for clinical training programs.

ASSESSING PHYSICIAN CARE

The recent focus on assessment of physician performance is being driven at least partially by financial concerns about how to reduce the costs of medical care. While various programs have been introduced to address rising health care costs (e.g., the implementation of a prospective payment system for Medicare and second-opinion programs), one of the greatest organizational changes that has occurred in recent years is the movement toward the reorganization of health care delivery from a fee-for-service system to a managed care environment.

The Managed Care Model

Most managed care programs, whether in the form of a preferred provider organization (PPO), a health maintenance organization (HMO), or an independent practice association (IPA), share a common concern for providing cost-effective patient care. The focal point of most managed care systems is the primary care physician, whose treatment and referral practices are believed to be a critical force in overall utilization patterns. Current medical school programs do little to prepare these practitioners for the level of scrutiny that will occur in their medical practices if they choose to participate in managed care programs.

Under managed care programs, the physicians' clinical credentials, their practice patterns, the environments in which they offer services, and in some instances their "commitment to a managed care philosophy" can be subject to review and evaluation. While specific review processes imposed on physicians will vary from one managed care program to another, an overview of the types of evaluations that can occur is provided here. The work of US Healthcare is used to highlight how some of these programs operate.[165,166] US Healthcare is an HMO whose subscribers are located primarily in the mid-Atlantic states.

Selection criteria for entry into US Healthcare (and most other managed care programs) constitute the first level of review the physician faces. This review can include a checklist related to whether the physician is board-certified, whether he or she has admitting privileges to one of the participating hospitals of the managed care program, and whether the physician or his or her group practice offers 24-hour coverage. In Donabedian's "structure-process-outcome" framework for assessing quality,[32] physician entry criteria for managed care programs tend to focus on the structural factors related to physicians' abilities to deliver health care services. In this manner, physicians' academic training that led to board certification can be directly tied to their abilities to receive hospital admitting privileges, and thus, their entry into certain managed care programs. The factors that are deemed to make a good office or practice environment, such as the number of examining rooms and the equipment for performing certain diagnostic tests, can also be part of the initial screen for selecting health care providers for an HMO. These entry criteria establish the essential building blocks for an acceptable practice environment, but they do little to ensure that high-quality care is delivered to the patients.

In addition to measuring the structural aspects of care, programs such as the one instituted by US Healthcare are designed to elicit patient feedback. This level of review includes an assessment of patient satisfaction with care, grievances, and requests for transfers to other primary care physicians. Under this type of system, quality of care evaluations of physician performance have been partially assigned to the patients. There is perhaps no better outcome of medical care available for assessment than how the patients regard the care they receive. These are not the types of tests that medical students and residents are accustomed to taking, and few physicians may be prepared to get this type of feedback once they are in practice. However, it would be feasible to link patient assessment of care into residency programs. While it is important that the senior resident evaluate the first-year resident's care, it may also be helpful to have the patients assess the quality of the care they have received. For the most part, the academic assessment of physician competence has been defined and measured by the profession. Other senior physicians determine what is high-quality and appropriate care. When the patients provide care assessments, as in some HMOs, measures of physician competence are expanded beyond what the profession is able to judge for itself.

Medical training programs may be able to build upon other evaluation processes used by managed care programs. As with peer review processes, many HMOs conduct periodic audits of medical records to examine certain standards of care. This might include an audit of the immunizations of children who have been seen by the physician or the evaluation of the use of mammography in women patients over 40 years of age. Diagnostic and treatment protocols are increasingly being used by managed care companies to conduct these types of chart review.

Health insurers and HMOs are in a unique position to evaluate physician performance since they receive detailed information on the services delivered to patients through the administrative data collected for payment purposes. In many ways, the databases of managed care and insurance companies contain a gold mine of information on the structure, process, and outcomes of care. These databases can be used to support programs that will lead to the continuous improvement of quality.

The Hospital Setting: Delineating Clinical Privileges

The delineation of clinical privileges is one of the most important means for hospitals to ensure high-quality care. The accurate assessment of a practitioner's clinical competence is one of the cornerstones of this process. Especially in light of today's turbulent environment of "new and powerful legal, health policy, economic and statutory forces, privilege delineation is increasingly important and requires sound information and leadership."[158] The American College of Physicians (ACP) has demonstrated such leadership by preparing guidelines for clinical competence in specific medical procedures under the auspices of the Clinical Privileges Project Steering Committee, a subcommittee of the College's Health and Public Policy Committee.[6]

Credentialing for procedures must be based on the expertise of the individual physician, not solely on "tickets" or certifying board examinations. The American Board of Internal Medicine (ABIM) certification, for example, will not ensure competence in the performance of the spectrum of procedures available for internists and the subspecialists of internal medicine.

Three equally important principles[67] are essential to all procedures and should be the basis of any learning and credentialing process: cognitive skills, technical skills (including manual dexterity), and the quality of the educators and the educational climate. The ACP guidelines for procedures such as percutaneous renal biopsy, endoscopic retrograde cholangiopancreatography (ERCP) and colonoscopy, for example, may outline: (1) a specific number of procedures to be performed; (2) an acceptable complication rate; and (3) a stipulated time period for completion of the procedure.

The ACP notes[6] that these guidelines are minimal suggested standards and their use does not abrogate the responsibility of the organization using them in making a final determination of physician competence. The guidelines are intended to be applied on a case-by-case basis in the context of well-defined privilege delineation and peer review processes. Finally, once a physician has established privileges in an institution, the guidelines will enable the institution to develop a reasonable approach to monitoring competence of individual physicians over their entire careers.

The work of the ACP in this area should serve as a bellwether for other representative groups within organized medicine. At minimum, academic training programs should make their trainees aware of the types of credentialing processes that are being defined by professional societies such as the ACP.

Review at the State Level

The peer review program of the Health Care Financing Administration (HCFA) is undergoing major changes. The traditional method of physician quality review under the PRO program targets single instances of quality problems. According to this system, quality problems are scored as a failure to meet existing quality standards. If the physician accumulates negative scores above the allowable level set by HCFA, a "corrective action plan" or sanctions may be imposed. This approach can be burdensome and expensive, and in essence, "keeps secret" from all but the reviewer the exact criteria used.

The DEMPAQ (Developing and Evaluating Methods to Promote Ambulatory Care Quality) project is a marked departure from the traditional PRO method of physician review. DEMPAQ,[104] a three-year demonstration project funded by HCFA and administered by Harvard University and the PROs of the State of Maryland and the District of Columbia, was created to develop an evaluative system for physician office care. DEMPAQ's philosophy rests with physicians' strong commitments among their peers for professional self-examination and self-improvement. The goal of the project is to spur physicians' efforts to improve their usual practices by enabling them, either as groups or as individuals, to compare their performances with those of their peers. DEMPAQ's computerized review system collects aggregate data on physician performances and feeds this information back to groups of physicians in the form of profiles and performance patterns. DEMPAQ "opens the 'black box' of quality criteria to physicians' scrutiny and evaluation."[78]

DEMPAQ consists of two review methods: Medicare claims profiling and medical record review. Review criteria based on quality indicators rather than on practice guidelines have been proposed for both sets of data. A computer algorithm is used to apply the review criteria to the data in order to generate profiles of physician practice. The American Medical Review Research Center (AMRRC)[7] is working with researchers to develop an educational package to accompany profiles that will be fed back to physicians, who in turn will critique the usefulness and relevance of this feedback.

The analysis of the Medicare claims involves structuring the data into patient-level profiles that describe physician practice patterns and performances. Three types of profile formats have been developed: office practice, condition-specific, and preventive care. The first format summarizes data about the physician's caseload, distribution of patient visits, and primary patient characteristics. The second format presents data for selected samples of patients with certain conditions and for use of services that contributes to good management of patients. This format also indicates the use of inefficacious or contraindicated types of care. The third format examines rates for certain preventive services (e.g., influenza immunizations, sigmoidoscopy, colonoscopy, Pap tests, and mammography for women).

The medical record review focuses on the adequacy of record documentation and performances of routine clinical functions such as testing, prescribing and monitoring drugs, procedures, and diagnosis. Record review criteria include seven common functions typically performed by the physician in the course of treating the patient: (1) responding to a complaint; (2) making a diagnosis; (3) ordering a test; (4) performing a procedure; (5) prescribing a drug; (6) following-up on serious health threats; and (7) providing prevention-screening services. For each of the seven functions, DEMPAQ has proposed a series of quality indicators that screen for activities that contribute to overall quality, rather than measure quality directly.

The DEMPAQ project and other ambulatory care review projects at the state level, such as the Wisconsin Ambulatory Review Project (WARP) and the Medicare Clinic Pilot Project, mark a discernible shift in the mode of physician review, from peer review to performance assessment.[112] Perhaps the most notable aspect of the DEMPAQ model is its proposed creation of a "normative curve" for ambulatory care practice patterns. While some element of clinical opinion is inherent in the peer-review process, and arguably should be, it is important for reviewers to have a barometer with which to gauge evaluation of physician performance.

CONCLUSION

We have described the early stages in the evolution of a national performance assessment system with examples from an HMO, the hospital setting, and the state level. What are the links between peer review and performance assessment vis-à-vis medical education, and can we develop additional innovative plans for the future in addition to the three presented here?

Both undergraduate and graduate medical education have contributed little to trainee understanding of and appreciation for the tools that are used to measure and improve the quality of medical care among practicing physicians. In addition, there is a dearth of appropriately prepared faculty, especially those with research credentials, available to teach the concepts of quality improvement and performance assessment. It is the exceptional residency program that includes discussions of quality improvement and resource utilization as an integral part of attending rounds and formal housestaff-oriented conferences.

Admittedly, medical education programs typically promote an apprentice system, where physicians are taught and evaluated by more senior clinicians. However, medical students can also gain by being evaluated by their patients and by their fellow students. The peer review process can be part of the educational system at the end of residency programs, because physicians should know how to review their peers and they should have had the experience of being the subject of review by their peers. In addition, physicians do not work in isolation; other members of the health care team should be involved in these types of feedback programs. For instance, an assessment by nurses of a resident's instructions should be part of the evaluation process. If physicians do not know whether their patients and other members of the health care team understood them, it will be a career-long struggle to be the team leader of the care delivered both in the hospital and in the outpatient setting.

In addition, medical education at all levels has been unable to directly tie the criteria for assessing the processes of care to patient outcomes. Simply, little pedagogic experience exists linking the environment of care (business school professors would call this the "organizational model") to patient mortality, for example. Other organizational design questions prompted by this type of analysis include analyzing the process of coronary bypass surgery and its relationship to surgical outcomes,[87] evaluating the organization of the medical staff and the quality of surgical care,[37] and the impact of intensive care unit staffing on the outcomes of patients with septic shock.[153] Perhaps training in these organizational issues will improve, enabling medical educators to establish a solid research foundation in this important field.

What of the future? O'Leary[135] believes that the "quality assessment tools of tomorrow will be reliable and valid performance measures, corresponding practice guidelines (or clinical standards or practice parameters), and reference databases that are carefully built from meaningful measures and guidelines. . . . It should be apparent that good performance data are the beginning rather than the conclusion of the quality assessment process . . . new analytic skills will prove to be essential ingredients in the new review activities."

Others recognize that improving the technology of peer review could bolster its validity and effectiveness.[168] Accomplishing this might include newer techniques for processing computerized information, electronic simulations for testing clinical judgments and skills, and the more widespread use of live simulations with standardized patients.[101] Segmenting the privilege-delineation process of the future by relying on a severity-adjusted credentialing process might also improve our ability to test performance criteria for clinicians.[116] It is likely that medical staffs would resist such efforts and a broad-based educational effort would be necessary to convince them of its utility.

Medical educators will no doubt play an expanded role in helping clinicians move away from traditional peer review toward performance assessment. Innovative programs to improve the quality of care, implemented by organizations such as HCFA,[82] may help stimulate this transition process. As performance evaluation systems for physicians in practice continue to grow, clinical training programs will be challenged to find ways to link these evaluation methods to academic medical programs.

CHAPTER FOUR

Assessment During Postgraduate Training

Jack Marshall, M.D.

One of the problems in comparing performance on graduation with performance in later years derives from the different objectives of training.

The undergraduate course tends in general to produce an undifferentiated doctor capable of being trained further in one of a number of specialist disciplines. Thus the educational process at the undergraduate level, with a few notable exceptions, tends to concentrate on the accumulation of detailed factual knowledge and is reflected by the use of multiple-choice questions in the major assessment process.

Course content in addition to the basic sciences concentrates on disease processes and body systems rather than on the patient as a whole, with little attention paid to the family unit and even less to the influence of the community.

McGuire[122] has defined the academic medical center's institutional mission, "to provide the right type of education and training for the requisite number and type of doctors, such that they will be able to function in the health care delivery system so as to manage effectively the health problems the population will face in the coming decade."

In general, the undergraduate assessment process within the hospital system tends to be summative, that is, end-point evaluation, with the main purpose of decision making usually being the assignment of pass or fail grades. Advantages of the summative process are that examiners can be selected and trained and standards can be monitored. Some disadvantages of this process, however, are that its artificial nature sacrifices validity for the reliability of multiple-choice items, little feedback about performances is given, the base of factual knowledge tends to be narrow, and many important aspects are difficult to assess. The major problem with summative assessment is that the assessment process determines the learning. Past examination papers are in greater demand than is patient contact.

Any review of the undergraduate curriculum should determine what behaviors are seen as desired at the point of graduation. The whole question of what skills should be present needs review. Little appears to have changed since the GPEP report[10] or the Edinburgh declaration.[34] Perhaps, as Bloom[15] stresses, the introduction of change is too difficult. Some of the problems related to assessment have been highlighted by Kane.[86]

UNDERGRADUATE LEVEL

At the undergraduate level, there has been, in general, little attempt to change the traditional assessment of essay questions, multiple-choice questions, and clinical examinations.

There is little doubt that multiple-choice questions are objective and very reliable. The main problem is that, to set a multiple-choice question the answer to which is not obvious, the question tends to be based on trivia rather than everyday problems. The pass mark is generally set at about 50–65%. It is unlikely that we would be happy with a graduate who had only 50% of the knowledge necessary to deal with a presenting problem.

The essay question in general has been unreliable; that marker variance between two markers can vary by as much as some 40% led the Royal Australian College of General Practitioners to abandon it many years ago. More recently the Royal College of General Practitioners also ceased using the traditional essay question.

The general management of the clinical case has often been assessed at a global level. Yet the clinical interview measures knowledge, interpretation, and problem solving as well as attitudes and communication skills. A global rating reveals little about the individual behaviors involved and can lead to the "halo" effect (i.e., good performance in one behavior may well mask poor performance in another).

A more recent innovation is the objective structured clinical examination (OSCE)[61] or objective structured clinical assessment (OSCA). In this test the candidate rotates through a series of stations, at each of which he is required to perform some task. Tasks may involve short-answer written questions, taking history from a patient, performing some procedural test, or interpreting data. This test is becoming more widely used, but, again, does not in general separate out the behaviors being measured, although it is certainly possible to do so.

A more comprehensive and more in-depth test has been developed at Southern Illinois University, where a series of standardized patients and an associated computer facility provide the entire assessment process.[191] The system can be used to assess knowledge, interpretation, problem solving, and interpersonal skills. This system, however, is unique to medical schools and no doubt has been difficult to achieve.

Many other schools have attempted to move from the traditional form of assessment, but with limited success. A major problem has been that graduates of such schools must compete with graduates of traditional schools for hospital posts and as such want to know how they compare with the students from the traditional schools. This has influenced the return of multiple-choice questions where initially such questions had not been seen as an appropriate test of competence.

Again, where national certifying examinations contain multiple-choice questions, students at innovative schools, where the curriculum is based on problem-based learning, spend their final few weeks attempting to learn factual knowledge from textbooks in order to pass the examinations. Unfortunately, the assessment system still tends to drive the learning process.

This diversity of assessment procedures at the undergraduate level makes comparison at a postgraduate level difficult, particularly if such assessment is directed at objective measurement of the skills necessary for competence in practice.

POSTGRADUATE LEVEL

At the postgraduate level, many colleges of physicians (e.g., the Royal Australian College of Physicians) have maintained an assessment process similar to that of medical schools, and it is not uncommon for postgraduate examinations to be conducted predominantly by using multiple-choice questions, often with up to six hours of testing time in any one day.

While summative assessment is not seen as ideal, there is unfortunately generally still a requirement to produce some summative evidence both to the public and to certifying bodies that competence has been achieved within the postgraduate training programs. In relation to the postgraduate training program for family practice in Australia, Abrahamson[1] recommended that "summative assessment should be introduced as an end point for training and possibly as an annual benchmark of achievement."

It may be possible to make the summative process more valid by thinking more laterally in terms of assessment tools and by facilitating the learning process by introducing formative assessment during the training period. Formative assessment has, as its aim, the identification of deficiencies during the training period in order to direct study to correct such deficiency. No pass-fail decision is made as a result, and the assessment process becomes constructive. Feedback related to deficiencies directs the learning program for each individual.

In its postgraduate training program, the Royal Australian College of General Practitioners makes extensive use of formative assessment and provides resources to enable trainees to take part in continuous self-assessment during the training period. This allows identification of deficient areas that can be addressed by using appropriate resource materials, also developed by the college.

As the fellowship examination is the end point of training, the formative assessment process attempts, as far as possible, to ensure that an adequate standard of competence has been attained prior to the formal, end-point (summative) assessment.

Learning is facilitated by replacing the lecture with small-group discussion and one-to-one interaction in the office with an experienced supervisor. When such a system is used, learning occurs rapidly, with each individual determining his or her own needs and identifying the resources required to meet them. No two individuals will have the same needs at any point in time, and each will progress at his or her own pace.

A MORE VALID PROCESS: AN EXAMPLE

To introduce appropriate summative assessment, it is necessary to define the anticipated outcomes of training. To look at a specific example, family practice has been defined by the Royal Australian College of General Practitioners as "the provision of primary, continuing, comprehensive, whole-patient care to individuals, families and their community":

1. *Primary* care implies the ability to accept responsibility for any presenting problem. In the management of a problem, referral may be made to other doctors, community services, or other health care professionals. Much of the work concerns ill-defined illness, and the practitioner frequently deals with problem complexes rather than specific diseases.

2. *Continuing* care implies an ongoing responsibility for the patient's health by applying the principles of prevention. Education of the patient to understand and to assume responsibility for his or her own health care needs is part of the process.
3. *Comprehensive* care implies decision making about health problems in all age groups and in all body systems as they affect the patient, taking note of the impact on the family and the general community.
4. *Whole-patient* care implies consideration of the whole person and the physical, psychological, social, and environmental factors that impact the patient.

What to Measure

To assess the abilities required by the competent family physician, one must define the elements that constitute the working day of the physician. These can be looked at in relation to the three domains of behavior defined by Bloom[14,96]:

1. *Cognitive*. This includes the important categories of (1) knowledge, not only of specific facts as measured by the multiple-choice question, but also knowledge of ways of organizing, studying, and judging these facts; (2) interpretation, which requires the comprehension of the data; and (3) problem solving, which analyzes the components of a problem and how they interrelate, allowing synthesis of the data to formulate a specific answer while excluding possible alternatives.
2. *Affective*. This domain is predominantly involved with behaviors related to values, interests, attitudes, emotional bias, and general philosophy. These behaviors have been classified as "receiving," "responding," "valuing," and "characterization"; they all pertain to a physician's interpersonal skills.
3. *Psychomotor*. This domain comprises perceptual and manual skills (e.g., those involved in the use of diagnostic instruments, surgical procedures, and resuscitation techniques).

Little attention has been paid in the undergraduate medical curriculum to teaching interpersonal or psychomotor skills. This may be a reflection of the fact that most teaching in medical school is performed by specialists who are themselves involved with particular body systems and neglect the concept of the patient as an individual.

The most powerful tool in teaching interpersonal skills is a videotape of the consultation which is time-consuming and requires considerable teacher expertise. While standardized patients may be used in assessing interpersonal skills, their use in teaching is limited by the lack of a visual record of the interview.

Competency-Based Assessment

To design an assessment process that covers all aspects considered necessary for competent family practice, various tests must be used, each designed to measure specific aspects of competence, that is, assessment must be competency-based.

Having determined the behaviors to be measured, the next step is to decide how important each behavior is in relation to the total assessment. In general, the majority of the physician's work is involved in problem solving and is influenced considerably by interpersonal (affective) skills. The assessment process should be designed to give appropriate recognition to this.

While it is understood that knowledge underlies all the behaviors, the actual recall of factual knowledge is not seen as the most important. Much stored knowledge is used automatically in interpreting and problem solving. However, any comprehensive assessment should include a broad sampling of knowledge related to the appropriate practice and at an appropriate level. In the past, much knowledge tested by multiple-choice questions was based on minutiae. Such questions are easier to construct and have more black-and-white answers. Facts that are recalled only very occasionally are probably better obtained from a recent text, particularly as what is valid today will be outdated tomorrow.

Weightings

Within the Royal Australian College of General Practitioners, a system of weightings has been developed that is thought to represent the importance of the behaviors in routine practice. The table of weightings is reconsidered from year to year, with a major review every five years.

From this consideration, the following weightings have been developed:

1. Cognitive skills, 66%:
   - A. Recall of factual knowledge, 14%
   - B. Interpretative skills, 18%
   - C. Problem solving, 34%
2. Affective (interpersonal) skills, 26%
3. Psychomotor (manual and perceptual) skills, 8%

Once the weightings have been decided, the test areas used to assess performance of the behaviors need to be addressed.

Tests Used

The tests used in the fellowship examination for the Royal Australian College of General Practitioners are of the following types: multiple-choice questions; clinical interpretation; patient management problems; diagnostic and management interviews involving role play (standardized patients); physical examination; practice assessment; and case commentary.

Each test is broken down into the behaviors measured by the specific test, as the candidate's performance is considered on the basis of the behavioral ratings rather than on each specific test area. This allows considerable breadth of assessment for each behavioral area, resulting in more confidence in the decision-making process related to performance.

Multiple-Choice Questions

The multiple-choice question examination in medicine was first applied as an assessment tool in 1955,[19] and was initially described in detail by Hubbard and Clemans.[74] This type of test is highly reliable and objective in measurement, although the validity of multiple-choice questions is often debatable. However, it is highly economical and can cover a wide range of topics in a short time. The staging of disease has also been used as a parameter in multiple-choice questions.[143]

Clinical Interpretation

Currently, clinical interpretation is being measured by an adaptation of the uncued-question (Un-Q) format developed at Jefferson Medical College.[188] In this test, a pictorial representation is accompanied by a related question giving background information on the material to be interpreted.

Patient-Management Problems

Patient-management problems are used to assess problem-solving ability. While difficulties with this type of assessment have been identified, these may in large part be due to difficulties in scoring.[117,118] Abrahamson[2] suggests that "a recent tendency to abandon this format of examination for psychometric reasons may yet be reversed with a little more study of scoring."

Diagnostic and Management Interviews

These tests are standardized-patient interviews, with the diagnostic interview being based on organic illness and the management interview on psychosocial problems.

Physical Examination

To test the ability to elicit physical signs, a series of problems is presented. One of six cases each year tests resuscitation skills, using a model.

Practice Assessment

Prior to the fellowship examination, each candidate submits a description of his or her practice and a log diary of 100 consecutive cases. An oral examination is carried out based on the material submitted.

Case Commentary

Case commentaries are submitted prior to the fellowship examination and are based on cases that reflect the candidate's knowledge of the patient in relation to the community setting and the ancillary services available.

It is important that the total assessment process is based on a breadth of content that accurately reflects the family physician's practice. A detailed account, including rating forms and illustrative examples, can be found in *The Assessment of Clinical Competence.*[36]

CONCLUSION

One of the problems in setting up an assessment to measure behaviors and, as a result, to identify specific deficiencies where these exist, is the relative complexity of the assessment, necessitating examiner training as well as regular review of the process. Such an assessment's major strength, however, is its ability to determine specific deficiencies, which can then be fed back to candidates in order that attention can be directed to improving standards.

Postgraduate assessment as determined by such a comprehensive process may make comparisons with undergraduate performance difficult, in that different and more specific qualities are being assessed than can be measured when relying purely on the multiple-choice questions, essay questions, and clinical oral examinations that still constitute most of the undergraduate assessment process.

CHAPTER FIVE

Relevance of "Irrelevant" Facts in Medical Education: The Value of Basic Science Teaching for Later Medical Practice (An Opinion Piece)

Wolfgang H. Vogel, Ph.D.

Many different components comprise a physician's performance. They include an individual's knowledge of medical facts and skills, a compassionate attitude towards the patient, long-term experience, fine communication skills, and other factors. Evaluation of the physician's performance will involve measurement or assessment of these components.[109] While these attributes are all important and significantly interact with each other, knowledge is perhaps the easiest to teach and to measure quantitatively. Thus, the accumulation of knowledge and its evaluation by examinations play major roles in medical education to prepare the student for a career in medicine and in the demonstration of a physician's competence in a given specialty. Performance is judged on the basis of retrieval of memorized theoretical and practical facts thought necessary to obtain a medical degree or to practice medicine.

In medical school, the education process consists of teaching these facts of medicine. Unfortunately, each discipline in the basic sciences and clinical specialities is convinced that it represents the most important part of medicine. Thus, the disciplines are likely to overwhelm young brains trying to cope with vast amounts of information by trying to convey all the knowledge that is available to them.[175] It is assumed that the more "relevant" facts the students know, the better physicians they will become. In fact, the relationship between performance measures in medical school and in practice can be described in terms of the relevance of the facts learned in medical school to their later application in the physician's practice. The quantity of facts learned becomes a main evaluator of the student and a predictor of future clinical performance. And, while the teachers turn on the spigots of information and the students struggle—and sometimes drown in the endless sea of wisdom, the students ask: (1) do we really have to learn all these facts?; (2) are they indeed necessary for us as practicing physicians?; and (3) can we not ease the onslaught by deleting the "irrelevant" and by concentrating on the "relevant" facts? These questions have been asked from the beginning of organized teaching by scores of panic-stricken students.

The terms *relevance* and *irrelevance* are extremely difficult to define, since they are relative. They depend largely on the knowledge available at a given time and on the orientation of the individual educator. As an example of the former, it was taught with authority in genetics only 50 years ago that proteins were extremely relevant because they formed the basis of life and that nucleic acids were rather irrelevant in this respect; today we know, of course, that the formerly irrelevant nucleic acids are the relevant building blocks of life and that the formerly relevant proteins, although quite important for many cellular mechanisms, are now relatively irrelevant from a genetic point of view. Here, current state-of-the-art and mainstream thinking determine what is relevant and what is irrelevant, a definition that can change quickly as research provides us with more pertinent information.

From the latter perspective, the definition rests with the educator and his or her opinion of what is relevant or irrelevant. The educator determines the information to be taught and tested. While some educators feel all facts are relevant (and, thus, overwhelm the students), others are selective (albeit not uniformly) in teaching relevant facts (perhaps omitting important and stressing unimportant information).

During our educational and professional careers, students and educators will never know what is relevant and what is irrelevant. Relevant facts may disappear and irrelevant facts may emerge as relevant as new information becomes available. The switching of the relevant to irrelevant and vice versa in the light of scientific advances affects the magnitude of relationships between facts learned in medical school and their implications in practice. The exact definitions of "relevance" and "irrelevance" rest solely in the brains of the beholders. Interestingly, too late to be of any use, there will be a time when we will definitively know what was relevant and what was irrelevant for each of us—at the end of our lives. Thus, truth lies in the individual's hindsight.

However, students do not yet have professional hindsight. They judge from the present and out of desperation learn to cope with seemingly unsurmountable amounts of facts, most of which seem trivial and unnecessary to them for their later lives. Of course, what they do not recognize yet is that many "relevant" facts will be of no practical importance to them while many "irrelevant" facts may become crucial in their future careers or may decide between the life and death of a patient. I remember a cartoon: as two ladies enter a room of an art museum filled with beautiful and priceless paintings, one points to a small, ordinary fire extinguisher in the corner and remarks that they must have been in this room before, since she remembers the fire extinguisher. How silly to forget the relevant beautiful paintings and to remember the irrelevant fire extinguisher—or perhaps not so silly in case of a fire. In a fire, this little, irrelevant piece of equipment could save all the beautiful, relevant works of art!

In spite of the reality that the students will learn more than they will ever use in their later lives, and yet not enough to be fully knowledgeable and prepared to start and continue their professional careers, this seemingly endless stream of information must serve another purpose as well. While we store all the relevant and irrelevant facts, we also train our brains to comprehend the information and to use it wisely. As we fit piece onto piece, we slowly construct a scientific and medical model until we begin to "see" the "Gestalt" of the human body in health and disease. Many facts taught as scientific truths eventually turned out to be completely wrong yet were instrumental in producing new, more accurate information and in advancing science. The true shape and course of the earth in the universe emerged from the concepts that the earth was flat and that the sun circled the earth—concepts once taught as relevant but later proven false were nevertheless a necessary step in creating today's relevant concepts.

Throughout history, "irrelevant" facts have evolved smoothly into relevant information in traditional ways or have been converted into better information by scientific revolutions, sometimes violently. Darwin started his famous voyage to collect biological information based on traditional scientific concepts that were then thought to be extremely relevant, though they are now known to be false. Since the facts he compiled did not fit the traditional mold, the "relevant" theories became irrelevant and were replaced with the better, now relevant hypothesis of evolution.

Thus, both "relevant" and "irrelevant" facts train our brains and allow us to better understand nature and life. They prepare us to comprehend the human body, to understand diseases, and to find new treatments. We can then develop more adequate theories, omit "wrong" information, add new facts, and improve our general knowledge. This general understanding allows us to advance science and medicine and to make rational decisions when the textbooks do not provide satisfactory answers.

The good educator bears a great responsibility. He or she must realize that certain facts are chiseled in granite and are absolutely relevant, and that certain other facts are soft and perhaps irrelevant. Nevertheless, not only the relevant information but also some of the irrelevant facts must be taught to help to elucidate general principles. In this context, "irrelevant" facts become relevant in spite of the fact that they are of no value taken alone. In the choice of "hard" or "soft" information to be presented, the educator must also keep in mind that the complete theoretical mixture of all of these facts greatly exceeds the capacity of the human brain. He or she must select, albeit on a very individual basis different from educator to educator and perhaps different on separate occasions by the same teacher, a core curriculum. Ideally, this core curriculum should fulfill two purposes: it should give the student a sufficient amount of hard information and knowledge necessary for his or her future career, and it should also give the student time to comprehend this wealth of material and to form general concepts. We expect the facts in the core curriculum to relate more to performance in practice than other "softer" facts.

Educators must not only update their own knowledge constantly but also communicate with other faculty members within their specialties and with those in other specialties of the school, as well as with practicing physicians, in order to obtain a reasonable compendium of "relevant" facts to be presented to the students. The students must concentrate and learn the material taught and not waste energy by agonizing over the relevance of the information. However, the students might later, as practicing physicians, also provide feedback to faculty members to make medical education more "relevant." This undertaking would have the potential to improve the education system by increasing uniformity, efficiency, and "relevance." The improved education system would significantly enhance the relevance of facts learned before graduation to later practice, allow for better predictions, reduce clinical mistakes, and improve patient care. The knowledge of "relevant" facts should correlate highly with their application in practice, at least in a juncture of time when those facts are still considered relevant.

PART THREE

Empirical Findings

If a thing exists, it exists in some amount.
If it exists in some amount, it can be measured.

Edward Lee Thorndike
1874–1949

CHAPTER SIX

The Relationship of Academic Measures in Medical School to Performance After Graduation

Ronald J. Markert, Ph.D.

Studies of the relationships between medical school academic predictors and outcome measures of physicians' performances have resulted in equivocal conclusions. Two reports published in the early 1970s, a book detailing two decades of research[147] and a literature review,[202] found little relationship between medical school grades and physicians' performances in practice. More recently, medical education researchers have investigated the association between a broad range of academic measures and assessment of effectiveness during residency. These researchers have found a significant, though moderate, relationship between performance in residency (usually the first year) and various medical school academic variables: grades,[35,45,89,98,186,206] clinical evaluations,[35,60,89,98,206] National Board of Medical Examiners (NBME) Part I examination scores,[24,45,159,184,186,206] NBME Part II scores,[45,60,89,159,184,186,206] and Alpha Omega Alpha membership.[35,98] Other studies have found scores on the postgraduate NBME Part III to be related modestly to medical school academic predictors: grades,[187] clinical evaluations,[20,187] and NBME Part I and Part II scores.[20,222,287] The relationship between medical school variables and performance after graduation is often lessened by the time gap between predictor and criterion and the differences among the constructs being measured.[114] The present study tested three research hypotheses:

1. Measures of medical school academic performance will correlate significantly with postgraduate outcome measures.
2. The relationship between measures of medical school academic performance and postgraduate outcomes will be strongest for measures that are conceptually similar.
3. Students who are categorized as being low or high academic performers in medical school will be categorized similarly on postgraduate outcome measures.

METHOD

The predictor set of medical school academic variables was preclinical grade-point average (GPA), clerkship GPA, NBME Part I total score, and NBME Part II total score. The clinical competence measures one year after graduation were NBME Part III total score and residency supervisor's rating. Graduates of Wright State University School of Medicine since its inception (classes of 1980 through 1991) participated in the study (n = 947).

Part III of the NBME examination is a measure of clinical competence at the level of the first-year resident and typically is completed by the resident late in the first postgraduate year. The physician supervisor rating form was developed at the University of Arizona.[30] The internal consistency reliability (Cronbach's alpha) of the physician supervisor rating form in this study was .964. The physician supervisor rating form was first used with the class of 1983, and thus data from this instrument were available for the classes of 1983 through 1991 (n = 801) only.

The Arizona form contains 18 scales: 11 scales yield ratings from 1 to 8: interpersonal skills with staff, interpersonal skills with patients, fund of medical knowledge, motivation/diligence, verbal and presentation skills, history-taking skills, physical examination skills, differential diagnosis/problem-listing skills, therapeutic planning, procedural skills, and overall evaluation; and seven scales yield ratings from 1 to 5: preparation at start of residency, resident's view of the preparation, understanding of goals and objectives of the residency, progress in learning and development during first year of residency, constructive use of feedback, use of educational resources of the residency program, and responsibility for own learning. Each of the 11 eight-point scales had five pertinent behavioral statements along the continuum. For example, on physical examination skills, a rater would mark a 1 or 2 if he or she agreed that the resident was "unable to perform an adequate physical exam; too often misses important findings." In contrast, a 7 or 8 would be assigned to the resident who fit the following description: "exceptionally skilled at physical examination; superior techniques, picked up things others missed." Each of the seven five-point scales had a germane behavioral description for each point on the continuum. For example, in rating the resident on use of educational resources, the physician supervisor would check 1 if the resident "used resources very ineffectively," and 5 if the resident "used resources very effectively."

Permission of the graduates was necessary to obtain NBME Part III scores and the physician supervisors' ratings. Of the 947 graduates from the classes of 1980 through 1991, 628 (66%) granted permission to obtain NBME Part III scores. Of the 801 graduates from the classes of 1983 through 1991, 481 (60%) granted permission to obtain their physician supervisors' ratings. Two preclinical GPAs were unavailable, hence sample sizes in regard to preclinical GPA and the two outcome measures were 626 and 480, respectively.

Pearson correlation and stepwise regression analysis (probability of F-to-enter=.05; no forced entry) were used to answer the first and second research hypotheses. Factor analysis with orthogonal varimax rotation and chi-square analysis were used to test the third research hypothesis.

RESULTS

The four medical school variables were significantly correlated with NBME Part III scores (n = 628) and physician supervisors' ratings (n = 481). Preclinical GPAs and clerkship GPAs were correlated .50 and .46 with NBME Part III scores. Not surprisingly, NBME Part I scores ($r = .56$) and NBME Part II scores ($r = .71$) were most highly correlated with NBME Part III scores. Medical school grades were moderately, though significantly, correlated with physician supervisors' ratings: .25 and .30 for preclinical GPAs and clerkship GPAs, respectively. NBME Part I and Part II correlations with physician supervisors' ratings were slightly lower: .20 and .24, respectively. All correlations were significant at $p < .001$.

The regression equation for NBME Part III scores accounted for 51% of the variance and consisted of three steps: NBME Part II scores (step 1: 50.3%), clerkship GPAs (step 2: 0.5%), and NBME Part I scores (step 3: 0.3%). Clerkship GPAs (step 1: 8.9%) and preclinical GPAs (step 2: 0.8%) entered the physician supervisors' ratings equation but accounted for only 10% of the variance. The correlation and regression analyses support the first two hypotheses: (1) medical school academic performance and postgraduate outcome measures are related; and (2) the relationships are strongest for conceptually similar measures.

Factor analysis of the four medical school academic variables resulted in one factor (eigenvalue = 2.97; percentage of variance = 74.4%). The factor loadings for the single-factor solution were: preclinical GPAs = .80, NBME I scores = .79, NBME II scores = .79, clerkship GPAs = .59). This factor was called *medical school academic achievement.*

Factor analysis of the 18-scale residency supervisor rating form yielded three factors with eigenvalues greater than one. The first factor (eigenvalue = 8.94; percentage of variance = 49.7%) was called *residency clinical competence* and was composed of seven scales that loaded .50 or greater (physical examination skills = .87, history-taking skills = .85, therapeutic planning = .75, differential diagnosis/problem listing skills = .72, verbal and presentation skills = .70, fund of medical knowledge = .53, and motivation/diligence = .50). The second factor (eigenvalue = 1.49; percentage of variance = 8.3%) was composed of six scales with .50 or greater factor loadings (resident's view of preparation = .77, preparation at start of residency = .71, understanding of goals and objectives of the residency = .70, overall evaluation = .68, interpersonal skills with staff = .63, and progress in learning and development during first year of residency = .50). The third factor (eigenvalue = 1.04; percentage of variance = 5.8%) contained three scales (use of educational resources of the residency program = .80, constructive use of feedback = .79, and responsibility for own learning = .65). The second and third factors combined accounted for only 14% of the variance and were not easily entitled. Thus, only the first factor was used in subsequent analyses.

Next, the predictor variable (i.e., the factor score indicating medical school academic achievement) was related to the two outcome criteria for the first year of residency (factor score for residency clinical competence and NBME Part III score). Study participants were divided into three groups on the three variables: top quarter, middle half, and bottom quarter. Tables 6.1 and 6.2 show these results.

Medical school academic achievement was significantly related to clinical competence in residency (Table 6.1) and NBME Part III scores (Table 6.2). For clinical competence in residency there was only a 13% probability of being in the top quarter if the graduate was in the bottom quarter in medical school academic achievement. Conversely, a graduate in the top quarter in medical school academic achievement had only a 13% probability of being in the bottom quarter of residency clinical competence. Even more pronounced were the results for medical school academic achievement and NBME Part III scores. Bottom-

Table 6.1 Relationship between Medical School Academic Achievement and Residency Clinical Competence for Three Categories of Graduates, 1983–1991, Wright State University School of Medicine

	Residency Clinical Competence							
	Bottom Quarter		Middle Half		Top Quarter		Total	
	No.	(%)	No.	(%)	No.	(%)	No.	(%)
Medical school academic achievement								
Bottom quarter	39	(42%)	41	(45%)	12	(13%)	92	(19%)
Middle half	64	(26%)	129	(51%)	58	(23%)	251	(52%)
Top quarter	18	(13%)	71	(52%)	48	(35%)	137	(29%)
TOTAL	121	(25%)	241	(50%)	118	(25%)		

$\chi^2 = 30.72$; df = 4; $p = < .0001$.

Table 6.2 Relationship between Medical School Academic Achievement and NBME Part III Score for Three Categories of Graduates, 1980–1991, Wright State University School of Medicine*

	NBME Part III Score							
	Bottom Quarter		Middle Half		Top Quarter		Total	
	No.	(%)	No.	(%)	No.	(%)	No.	(%)
Medical school academic achievement								
Bottom quarter	71	(62%)	41	(36%)	2	(2%)	114	(18%)
Middle half	84	(26%)	200	(61%)	45	(14%)	329	(53%)
Top quarter	5	(3%)	67	(37%)	111	(61%)	183	(29%)
TOTAL	160	(26%)	308	(49%)	158	(25%)		

$\chi^2 = 249.67$; df = 4; $p = < .0001$.

* NBME = National Board of Medical Examiners

quarter medical school achievers had only a 2% probability of being in the top quarter for NBME Part III scores, and top-quarter medical school achievers were only 3% likely to be in the bottom quarter for NBME Part III scores. These results support the third hypothesis: students who are categorized as being low or high academic performers in medical school will be categorized similarly as first-year residents.

DISCUSSION

The predictive validity of medical school academic variables was examined by using measures from the first year of residency as the criteria. Medical school grades and scores on NBME Parts I and II were significant predictors of NBME Part III scores and physician supervisors' ratings, with correlations ranging from .20 to .71. Chi-square analysis using factor-analysis-derived variables substantiated the ability of medical school academic achievement to predict residency clinical competence and NBME Part III scores.

Not unexpectedly, measures closer in construct to the criterion had greater predictive validity. For example, the highest correlations were between scores on NBME Parts I and II and scores on NBME Part III. Furthermore, the highest correlation with physician supervisors' ratings among the medical school academic variables was with clerkship GPAs ($r = .30$), perhaps due to the inclusion of physician preceptor ratings of the medical student as a component of each clerkship grade. When the criterion is less conceptually similar to the predictor, relationships are not as impressive. The limited predictive validity of medical school variables for residency performance in the first year of postgraduate education as measured by physician supervisors' ratings is demonstrated by a regression equation that accounts for only 10% of the variance.

To examine the effect of response rate, the *t*-test was used to compare the performances on the medical school academic variables of those graduates who did and those who did not grant permission to use their outcome measures. Consenting graduates (for NBME Part III scores or physician supervisors' ratings) differed from non-consenting graduates (no NBME Part III scores or no physician supervisors' ratings) in nearly all cases. For all four measures, consenting graduates (for NBME Part III scores) had significantly higher medical school academic performances ($p < .001$). For all but preclinical GPAs, consenting graduates (for physician supervisors' ratings) had significantly higher scores ($p < .005$). Thus, restriction of range in the present study may have caused the statistical relationships to be underestimates of the population. Consenting and nonconsenting graduates did not differ on the demographic variables of age (*t*-test) and gender (chi-square test).

The ability of medical school variables to correlate with a clinical postgraduate criterion is limited if the criterion is unreliable or lacks variability (usually due to a pronounced tendency for raters to assign high scores). The internal consistency reliability in the current study was impressive (.964). The mean score for physician supervisors' ratings was 93, with 123 being the maximum (standard deviation = 14.2). Thus, physician supervisors were rating residents reliably and with only a minimal tendency toward a ceiling effect.

This study demonstrates that medical school variables (preclinical GPAs, clerkship GPAs, and scores on NBME Parts I and II) have reasonable predictive validity, more so for NBME Part III scores than for physician supervisors' ratings. This study provides information about the predictive validity of traditional medical school measures. Also, the findings can be used in comparative studies in which recent and future changes in the examinations of the NBME[26] (now called United States Medical Licensing Examination) are investigated. Replications of this study at other medical schools would be especially useful in clarifying the relationships between predictors and criteria used in medical education.

CHAPTER SEVEN

The Empirical Association Between Student and Resident Physician Performances

Louise Arnold, Ph.D., and T. Lee Willoughby, M.S.

The relationship between performance in medical school and performance in residency has been a topic of enduring interest for research in medical education. Early studies indicated little association between performance of graduate physicians and premedical grades, Medical College Admission Test (MCAT) scores, medical school admission interview ratings, and medical school grades.[156,202] Since publication of that work three decades ago, researchers in this area have typically concluded that at best "there are low but statistically significant relationships between measures of medical school achievement and ratings of residency performance."[206]

At the same time, effort has been devoted toward increasing the ability to predict graduate physicians' performances from medical school achievements. Although many methodologic problems attend this effort,[203] several steps have been taken to enhance the understanding of the nature of the linkage between the medical school achievements and graduate performances of physicians. One approach, addressing the skewed nature of residency performance ratings,[186] has used distribution-free statistics, rather than the more frequently encountered parametric statistics, to examine that linkage.[45] Another approach has sought to maximize the relationship between medical school achievement and graduate performance by developing distinct components or dimensions of performance and examining the strengths of associations between like and unlike components. For example, when factors derived from medical school performance measures were correlated with several indicators of residency performance, relatively strong relationships were obtained between the factor labelled "National Board of Medical Examiners Part I" and specialty board scores, and between factors labelled "faculty evaluations" and "academic distinction" in medical school, on the one hand, and in-training residency performance evaluations, on the other.[28]

The authors of the present study have combined these two approaches in an effort to test them on another database and thereby increase the understanding of the relationship between medical school achievements and performances in residency. Their previous work in this area used correlational analysis with potentially heterogeneous measures of: (1) performances of students in a combined baccalaureate-MD degree program; and (2) these students' subsequent performances in residency. Accordingly, the authors investigated the following questions:

- Are the categories of students' performance levels in the combined-degree program directly and significantly associated with their respective standings on clinical performance ratings as residents?
- Is this association between performances in the combined-degree program and residency stronger for those measurements that are conceptually more similar than dissimilar?

METHOD

The study group for this research was formed from the population of the 336 students who entered a six-year baccalaureate-MD degree program in 1980 through 1983 at the University of Missouri–Kansas City School of Medicine and who graduated. Of these graduates, 298 (89%) constituted the study group, because complete records of their baccalaureate degree work, medical school achievements, and clinical performances in the first year of residency training were available.

Measures of Student Performance

Grades, test scores, and clinical performance evaluations that the study group received while completing the curricular components of the combined-degree program constituted the 16 measures of student performance used in this research.

More specifically, the authors used the cumulative grade-point average (GPA) each student earned in courses for the baccalaureate degree.

The GPA included grades for liberal arts courses, premedical-school courses in chemistry, anatomy, microbiology, and such biology electives as genetics and medical-school-level courses in physiology, biochemistry, and microbiology. The highest possible GPA was 4.0.

Test scores reflected students' performances expressed as percentages of questions answered correctly on the in-house quarterly profile examinations (QPEs). These comprehensive examinations were designed as longitudinal measures of students' acquisition and retention of knowledge in the basic and clinical sciences of medicine. The authors used total scores the individual students achieved on the QPEs taken during the fifth year of the curriculum. The QPEs are reliable and valid measures of students' knowledge of basic and clinical sciences.[201] Pearson correlation coefficients reflecting the association between students' QPE scores and their scores on Parts I and II of the examinations of the National Board of Medical Examiners (NBME) have ranged from .7 to .8 in the past. Because of the strength of these correlations, QPE scores can be viewed as proxies for NBME examination scores, which were not available for all 298 study group participants.

The clinical performance evaluations (CPEs) were based on the mean ratings instructors gave students in 11 required clinical rotations in years three through six of the curriculum. The rotations represented all the major areas of clinical medicine. Four of these rotations occurred in internal medicine, which all students took annually during the last four years of the curriculum as members of health care teams, usually under the supervision of the same instructors, called docents, for these rotations. The CPEs provided a means of collecting data from instructors about the students' attitudes, peer relations, reliability, knowledge of medical information, concepts, skills, maturity, rapport with patients, ingenuity, conscientiousness, and integrity. Behavioral descriptions of these dimensions were provided to the instructors to increase consistency across raters as they used a nine-point scale to assess students.

Measures of Graduate Performance

Ratings that the residents in the study group were given for their clinical performances by their residency supervisors at the close of their first postgraduate year constituted the measure of graduate performance used in this study. These ratings were taken from the school's annual follow-up survey of its graduates. Each graduate was rated along a seven-point scale in nine categories of clinical performance.

Defined by descriptive behaviors, these categories were problem-solving ability, independent learning ability, critical thinking ability, self-assessment ability, clinical skills, rapport with patients, relationships with colleagues, ability to work in groups, and professional responsibility. Although two of these categories (professional responsibility and clinical skills) contained behaviors regarding the graduates' funds of knowledge, the survey of residency performance was purposefully designed to highlight graduates' attributes other than their knowledge bases. Knowledge, it was reasoned, could best be ascertained through national standardized examinations. However, because the graduates' scores on the NBME III were not available for the entire study group, they were not examined in the present study.

Graduates of the school were asked at the end of their final year, or six months into residency if necessary, to give permission to gather information about their residency performances.

The specialty areas that the graduates entered for the first year of residency training were also included in the database.

Procedures

Components of Performances in the Combined-Degree Program

Data on the study group's performances during the combined-degree program were subjected to factor analysis. This technique was used to generate a parsimonious set of performance measures more manageable for subsequent analysis of the relationship between performances as students and as residents. More important, it was used to produce measures so that each would index similar performances distinct from other performances. Principal-component factor analysis was applied initially to the data and was followed, where appropriate, by orthogonal varimax rotation procedures to simplify the obtained factor structures.

The factor analysis of the 16 measures of performance in the combined-degree program yielded four initial factors with eigenvalues greater than unity. The orthogonal varimax rotation procedure resulted in the following factors and factor loadings. Factor I represented the GPAs and the four individual QPEs of the study group. All of these measures had factor loadings greater than .50; the highest loading equaled .85 for the February QPE and the lowest loading equaled .79 for the May QPE. No other performance measure correlated .50 or higher with this factor. Factor I was thus entitled *knowledge*. Factor II represented the CPEs obtained for the study group from the four internal medicine rotations. All of these measures had factor loadings greater than .50; the highest loading was .85 for the year-four rotation and the lowest was .50 for the year-six rotation. No other performance measure correlated .50 or higher with this factor. Accordingly, Factor II was labeled *internal medicine performance.* Factor III represented the CPEs obtained for the study group from required rotations in pediatrics, obstetrics-gynecology, surgery, and emergency medicine. All of these measures had factor loadings greater than .50; the highest loading was .65 for pediatrics and the lowest was .51 for obstetrics-gynecology. No other performance measure had a factor loading of .50 or higher. Thus, Factor III was labelled *other clinical sciences performance.* Factor IV concerned only the required psychiatric rotation, with a factor loading of .83. This factor was called *psychiatry performance.*

These four factors were defined, then, as the major components of performance in the combined-degree program; and a composite performance score for each of the four components was calculated for each student in the study group.

Components of Graduate Performances

The ratings the students received as graduates in nine areas of clinical performance during the first year of residency training were also factor-analyzed. Based on previous research, it was anticipated that four factors would emerge: knowledge and intellectual abilities, technical skills related to data gathering, relations with patients, and relations with colleagues and other health professionals.[8] However, the present analysis resulted in a one-factor solution with an eigenvalue greater than unity. Each of the nine areas had a factor loading greater than .50. The largest loading was .89 for clinical skills and the smallest was .79 for rapport with patients.

A composite score for this "grand factor," or *residency clinical performance* component, was derived for each study participant from the mean of the ratings each was given in the nine areas of performance by the residency supervisor.

Performance Levels

The resultant scores for performances during the combined-degree program and residency were rank-ordered for the individual components. Three categories were formed from the *residency clinical performance* ranking: *low,* representing the bottom 18% of the study group, whose mean ratings ranged from 1.5 to 4.9; *mid,* covering the middle 56% of the group, with mean ratings from 5.0 to 6.4; and *high,* representing the top 26%, with mean ratings from 6.5 to 7.0. These cutting points were selected by taking into account the distributions of the ratings awarded and the meanings of the labels assigned to the numerical-scale points used in the survey. The same categories of performances were created from the rankings of performance in the combined-degree program: low, representing the bottom 18% of the scores; mid, covering the middle 56% of the scores; and high, covering the top 26%.

These performance levels were used in subsequent analysis of the relationship between performances of the study group as students and then as residents.

Analysis of the Relationship Between Student and Graduate Performances

Because the distributions of performance ratings were skewed, the authors used nonparametric statistical methods to ascertain the association between the performances of the study participants as students and as resident physicians. They constructed contingency tables to relate the participants' performance levels on each of the four components of student performance (*knowledge, internal medicine performance, other clinical sciences performance, and psychiatry performance*) to their performance levels on the one *residency clinical performance* component.

They then subjected the data to chi-square analysis to gain answers to the research questions stated at the outset of the paper. The authors hypothesized that the *knowledge* component of performance in the combined-degree program would be less strongly related to the *residency clinical performance* component than would the clinical performance components based on evaluations from medical school rotations in the combined-degree program. They anticipated that the *internal medicine performance* component of performance in the combined-degree program would bear the strongest relation to *residency clinical performance* because of prior research results[89] and because of the program's academic plan. According to that plan, the ratings students receive in internal medicine are typically assigned by physicians who supervise the same students for four annual rotations of two months duration each and for four years of weekly outpatient clinic service. Thus, the authors also expected that the *internal medicine performance* component would continue to bear the strongest association with *residency clinical performance* when they introduced the specialty area of the graduates as a control factor, despite other work that had found that relationships between medical school achievement and graduate performance depended upon the specialty areas students entered as resident physicians.[28]

Standard computer procedures were used for the data analysis.[164]

RESULTS

To what extent were the categories of students' performance levels in the combined-degree program directly and significantly associated with their respective standings on clinical performance ratings as residency physicians? On average, 45% of the study participants were in the same performance categories as students and as residents. The largest proportions (from half to almost two-thirds) of the study participants in identical performance categories as students and as residents were those at the mid levels of performance. The smallest percentages (from about one-tenth to one-fourth) of participants in identical student and residency performance categories were those in the low performance-level groups.

Of special interest is the agreement between high and low levels of student and residency performance, respectively. In this regard, the most congruence was obtained with the component of *other clinical sciences performance* in the combined-degree program. The agreement was evident at both ends of the performance spectrum. That is, 42% of the participants in the high group of the *other clinical sciences performance* component were also in the high group of the *residency clinical performance* component, and 27% who were in the low group of the other *clinical sciences* component placed in the low group of *residency clinical performance.* The *internal medicine performance* component in the combined-degree program had the least agreement across the high levels of performance components. The *psychiatry performance* component had the least agreement between low performance categories.

Tables 7.1 through 7.4 present data bearing on the associations between the individual components of student performance in the combined-degree program and the *clinical performance* component in residency. The data did not entirely support expectations that a relationship between dissimilar performance components, such as that between *knowledge* and the *residency clinical performance* rating, would be weaker than a relationship between similar performance components. Each component of performance in the combined-degree program, including *knowledge* (Table 7.1), was associated with the residency component at a statistically significant level. The *other clinical sciences performance* component (Table 7.2), not the *internal medicine performance* component (Table 7.3), had the strongest association with the *residency clinical performance* component; the contingency coefficient was .27, the chi-square was 23.456, and the p level was highly significant ($< .001$). The *knowledge* component as well as the *internal medicine* and *psychiatry* components (Table 7.4) were each similarly associated with the *residency clinical performance* component. The contingency coefficients were .18; the chi-squares were 9.942, 9.748, and 10.272, respectively; and the *p*-values were .04, .05, and .04, respectively.

The degrees of association between components of performance in the combined-degree program and in residency when controlled for specialty area could not be examined by chi-square analysis. Too many cells in the contingency tables had less than adequate expected counts.

DISCUSSION AND CONCLUSIONS

On average, nearly half of the study participants were in the same performance categories as students in the combined-degree program and as residents. Half to almost two-thirds of the study participants who were in the mid levels of performance as students placed similarly on the *residency clinical performance* component in the mid category. However, the extent of agreement between the high and low performance standings of study participants as students and as residents is of most interest. At best, the proportion of study participants who fell into the same extreme categories of performance as students and as residents reached 42% among the high group. The greatest agreement between the student and residency components at the extremes of performance was obtained when the *other clinical sciences* component was examined against residency performance. The least agreement at the extremes was found when the *psychiatry* component was studied in relation to residency performance; only 11% of the low group of this component subsequently placed in the low group of the residency component.

The proportion of participants in the low performance groups during the combined-degree program and again in residency amounted to a little more than one-fourth. This relatively small proportion deserves comment. The clinical performance rating forms used in this study, both in the combined-degree program and at the graduate level, neither instructed supervisors to identify "weak" learners nor instructed them to assign students or residents to high or low performance categories. Rather, the forms asked them to rate learners by using behaviorally anchored scales. Perhaps if the forms had explicitly requested supervisors to identify weak learners, the agreement between performance standings in the combined-degree program and in residency would have been greater. The lack of such explicitness in the forms could explain the stronger associations obtained by other investigators whose graduate performance instrument required supervisors to place residents into quartiles.[45] It is, of course, the weak student

Table 7.1 Numbers and Percentages of 298 Graduates at Three Levels of *Knowledge* as Students and Three Levels of *Clinical Performance* as Residents, Entering Classes of 1980–1983, Baccalaureate-MD Program, University of Missouri–Kansas City School of Medicine

Level of *Clinical Performance* as Residents	Level of *Knowledge* as Students: High		Mid		Low	
	No.	%	No.	%*	No.	%
High	31	36	35	22	12	22
Mid	45	53	93	58	28	52
Low	9	11	31	19	14	26

$\chi^2 = 9.942$; df = 4; $p = .04$.
*Column total does not equal 100% because of rounding.

Table 7.2 Numbers and Percentages of 298 Graduates at Three Levels of *Other Clinical Sciences Performance* as Students and Three Levels of *Clinical Performance* as Residents, Entering Classes of 1980–1983, Baccalaureate-MD Program, University of Missouri–Kansas City School of Medicine

Level of *Clinical Performance* as Residents	Level of *Other Clinical Sciences Performance* as Students: High		Mid		Low	
	No.	%	No.	%	No.	%
High	33	42	39	23	6	12
Mid	41	53	94	56	31	61
Low	4	5	36	21	14	27

$\chi^2 = 23.456$; df = 4; $p = <.001$.

Table 7.3 Numbers and Percentages of 298 Graduates at Three Levels of *Internal Medicine Performance* as Students and Three Levels of *Clinical Performance* as Residents, Entering Classes of 1980–1983, Baccalaureate-MD Program, University of Missouri–Kansas City School of Medicine

Level of *Clinical Performance* as Residents	Level of *Internal Medicine Performance* as Students: High		Mid		Low	
	No.	%	No.	%	No.	%
High	22	30	47	28	9	16
Mid	46	62	86	51	34	61
Low	6	8	35	21	13	23

$\chi^2 = 9.748$; df = 4; $p = .05$.

Table 7.4 Numbers and Percentages of 298 Graduates at Three Levels of *Psychiatry Performance* as Students and Three Levels of *Clinical Performance* as Residents, Entering Classes of 1980–1983, Baccalaureate-MD Program, University of Missouri–Kansas City School of Medicine

Level of *Clinical Performance* as Residents	Level of *Psychiatry Performance* as Students: High		Mid		Low	
	No.	%	No.	%	No.	%
High	29	37	34	21	15	28
Mid	34	43	99	60	33	61
Low	16	20	32	19	6	11

$\chi^2 = 10.272$; df = 4; $p = .04$.

and the weak graduate who are in most need of correct identification for remediation or perhaps dismissal.

In the present study, each of the components of performance in the combined-degree program was associated with the residency component at a very modest, but statistically significant, level. This result echoes the conclusions reached by other investigators, despite the fact that it is based on distribution-free statistics and on purportedly cleaner and more homogeneous measures of performance.

Why were the associations not stronger? Performances of some study participants may have changed over the courses of their student and graduate careers. Measurement errors might well attenuate the student and graduate performance relationship. The use of newer methods to measure clinical performance more objectively[141] might have yielded more robust results, although those methods can be narrowly focused. Too, the number of study participants was relatively small for chi-square analysis. Further, the factor analysis of the ratings of residents' clinical performances did not yield distinct dimensions, as in the authors' prior work. A change in the format of the form that was used in this research might account for this result. Alternatively, perhaps residency supervisors were not able to discriminate between performance areas, as noted in a study of the American Board of Internal Medicine resident evaluation form.[180] That the factor analysis did not yield distinct components might approximate more closely the actual state of evaluations that measure performance in residencies. Yet, if the factor analysis had successfully identified components of the residency ratings, stronger associations between like components might have emerged. Some support for this speculation lies in the pattern of single-order correlation coefficients obtained in this data set between GPA and several QPEs, on the one hand, and residency performance ratings in each of the nine areas, on the other. These performance indicators of student knowledge tended to be related to those graduate areas that contained references to knowledge, such as clinical skills, or to such higher-order intellectual abilities as problem solving and critical thinking. The correlation coefficients ranged from .13 to .30, with p-values from .03 to $<.001$.

The strongest association in the present work, however, was indeed found between a component of student performance in clinical rotations and the *residency clinical performance* component. This result coincides with published[110] and unpublished results the authors have consistently obtained across data sets. In the present work, the *other clinical sciences* component (based on student performances in surgery, emergency medicine, pediatrics, and obstetrics-gynecology) was the strongest correlate of *residency clinical performance* and exhibited the greatest agreement across the low performance categories. Perhaps this empirical association reflects the context in which these performance assessments are made at the school. Instructors in these areas see students over the course of a two-month clerkship only. Nevertheless they interact with virtually all students in a class and are recognized by the promotion committee for their candor in identifying students who are clinically weak. In contrast, the *internal medicine* component is derived from assessments that docents make of student performances over four years. Although this relationship theoretically enhances the docents' ability to assess students, each docent observes only a fraction of the students in any one class. Further, the relationship between a docent and student is ongoing and may encourage docents to value, perhaps overvalue, their students' strengths.

Other contextual variables that were not examined here could have also contributed to the present results. These include the emphasis accorded clinical education in the combined-degree program that the study participants attended, the participants' specialty areas, and the quality of their residencies. However, through a proxy measure of program quality, namely degree of program affiliation with a university medical center, the authors endeavored to examine the relationship between quality of residency and ratings given to graduates. A cross-tabulation revealed that the degree of a program's affiliation with a university was not associated with the level of performance achieved by the school's graduates ($n = 289$, chi-square = 6.599, $p = .580$).

In another study of the relationship between medical school achievement and clinical performance in residency, the present authors concluded that the most reasonable means of predicting students' performances as residents might be to supplement medical school performance assessments with information about students' personal qualities.[110] The suggestion stems from a research record in which the strongest associations between student and graduate performances were obtained by using a combination of students' personal characteristics and their cognitive and noncognitive achievements in medical school.[68,89,90] Perhaps the absence of information about these personal characteristics of study participants also contributed to the present study's modest results. Finally, it could be that the strength of empirical relationships between performances in medical school and in residency are inherently limited because performances expected in residencies may not be mere extensions of those expected of students in medical school.

CHAPTER EIGHT

Clinical Performance-Based Test Sensitivity and Specificity in Predicting First-Year Residency Performance

Nu V. Vu, Ph.D., Linda H. Distlehorst, Ph.D., Steven J. Verhulst, Ph.D., and Jerry A. Colliver, Ph.D.

Clinical examinations based on standardized patients have recently been developed and adopted by medical schools and certification boards to derive more direct assessments of examinees' clinical skills and competence.[55,131,140,154,162,173,174,191,199] The design and development of this new assessment method arose mainly from the limitations often observed with existing ones, such as written examinations and direct observation of examinees' performances in actual clinical situations. With written examinations, examinees are at best assessed on their knowledge and on what they say they will do in a clinical encounter instead of what they actually do. On the other hand, with observation of examinees' performances, the main problems reside in the infrequency of observations of students by faculty,[169,174] the limited availability of and lack of standardization of patient problem presentations, and the subjectivity and variability of faculty ratings of students' performances.

In clinical examinations based on standardized patients,[55,131,140,154,162,173,174,191,199] examinees typically encounter a number of patient problems, each simulated by a standardized patient, a person carefully coached by a specific training method to accurately portray an actual patient.[11] With each problem the examinees are assessed directly on their interactions with and workups of the patient, namely, on their ability to perform a history and physical examination, to educate the patient, and/or to interact with and relate to the patient. In most testing situations, the examinees are also given a follow-up written test to assess their skills in evaluating the patient's problems, in ordering relevant laboratory and diagnostic tests, in interpreting the test results, and/or in managing the patient.[55,131,140,154,162,173,174,191,199] Until now, these examinations have been used mainly to determine examinees' levels of clinical performance, and very rarely for the purpose of certification for practice or promotion to the next level of training.[55,154,162,191,199] At our institution, the Southern Illinois University School of Medicine, a postclerkship examination (PCX) based on standardized patients has been administered every year for the last seven years (1986–1992) to all fourth-year medical students at the end of their clerkship rotations in order to assess their readiness for residency training.[191,199] Since satisfactory performance on the PCX is one of the requirements towards graduation, students' scores on the examination are interpreted in reference to the examination's satisfactory standard, or cutoff score, which is set by the faculty. When students' scores are above or below the cutoff score they are considered to be achieving or not achieving the required level of competence, hence being satisfactory or unsatisfactory, and ready or not ready for residency training. Given that this type of examination is relatively new and few applications have been intended for promotion and certification purposes, existing data supporting the validity of its use to make promotion and certification decisions are limited.[162]

The purpose of our study was to assess the utility of the PCX, a measure of students' clinical performances in the senior year, in predicting their first-year residency performance ratings. Distribution-free statistical methods were used in this study because of the common findings of skewness and restriction of range in the residency performance rating distributions[186,204] and the effects of these factors on the results derived from correlational studies using the Pearson product-moment correlation.[23,59,69] More specifically, the study assessed: (1) the PCX's sensitivity, that is, its ability to identify correctly those students who would receive high performance ratings in residency; (2) the PCX's specificity, that is, its ability to identify correctly those students who would not receive high ratings in residency; (3) the rates of false negatives and false positives obtained when using the PCX; and (4) the PCX's predictive values, that is, its ability to determine the probability that a student with a satisfactory or unsatisfactory performance on the PCX would receive a high or low rating in residency, respectively.

METHOD

Participants

This study was based on the PCX scores of the classes of 1987 ($n = 67$), 1988 ($n = 69$), and 1990 ($n = 66$) and their first-year residency supervisors' ratings. Sixty-three percent ($n = 42$) of the 1987 Class, 78% ($n = 49$) of the 1988 class, and 77% ($n = 51$) of the 1990 class gave the institution permission to collect data from the supervisors of their postgraduate training programs. Two classes were not included in the study: the class of 1986 because the students' scores on the 1986 PCX, the first to be administered, were calculated differently from those in subsequent years; and the class of 1989 because of the low permission rate for follow-up obtained for that class (35%).

Instrument

Postclerkship Examination (PCX)

Students' performances on the PCX of 1987, 1988, and 1990 was based on 17,17, and 18 patient cases, respectively. For most of the cases, students had a 20-minute encounter with the standardized patient followed by a 20-minute written test. In the patient encounter, the students were assessed on their abilities to perform a relevant history, physical examination, and/or patient education, and to communicate with and relate to the patient. On the written test, they were assessed on their abilities to indicate the relevant history and physical examination findings, to formulate the working and final diagnoses, to order laboratory and diagnostic procedures, to interpret the results of the procedures, and to plan the management for the patient. The students' performances on the PCX were reported by two scores: the clinical competence score (CCS), which reflects performances on all of the above-mentioned abilities except those of communicating and relating to the patient; and the professional behavior score, which reflects performances on the two latter abilities. The use of two separate scores in reporting students' performances on the PCX had been confirmed in an earlier-analytic study[192] that showed that the PCXs consistently assessed two separate factors or skills: a cognitive skill (similar to the CCS) and a noncognitive one (similar to the professional behavior score). The classification of satisfactory or unsatisfactory performance on the PCX was based solely on the CCS and not on the professional behavior score, which has been used only for the purpose or identifying and counseling students who received low professional and patient-satisfaction ratings. For these reasons, only the CCSs are used in this study to assess the utility of the PCX in predicting supervisors' ratings of students' performances in their first year of residency.

Students' CCSs on the PCXs of 1987, 1988, and 1990 ranged from 54 to 77 of a possible 100, with a mean of 70; from 60 to 75, with a mean of 69; and from 57 to 77, with a mean of 71, respectively. A student was considered to achieve satisfactory or unsatisfactory performance on the PCX when his or her CCS was higher or lower, respectively, than the satisfactory-performance standard, or cutoff score, set for the examination. The PCX cutoff score is criterion-referenced and is the average of all the cutoff scores for the individual cases on the PCX. For each case on the PCX, a case cutoff score is set, representing the minimal criterion or score that faculty have agreed a student should obtain in order to be considered to perform satisfactorily on that case. A detailed description of the PCX, presented earlier,[191] should be referred to for a full description of the examination and of its scoring and cutoff score setting. The cutoff scores derived for the PCXs of 1987,1988, and 1990 were 66, 65, and 69, respectively. It should be noted that because the PCX was administered at the end of the students' clinical clerkship rotations, their performances on the PCX were not registered on their transcripts at the time of their residency applications and hence not known to the residencies at the time of their interviews.

First-Year Residency Supervisors' Ratings

As part of the university's longitudinal assessment effort, graduates' clinical performances are assessed at the end of their first postgraduate year. Through a questionnaire, residency supervisors are asked to assess the graduates' performances in 13 areas on a ten-point rating scale (10 = outstanding; 9–8 = above average; 7–4 = satisfactory; 3–2 = below average; and 1 = unsatisfactory).[136]

Like the results obtained with the PCX factor analyses, the results of factor-analytic studies of the supervisors' ratings showed that two main factors or dimensions were assessed by the ratings.[94,189] The first was the clinical competence ratings (CCR), which is the average of the ratings for eight areas: history taking, physical examination, problem identification, diagnostic approach, management, general knowledge, independent learning, and technical skills. The second was the professional behavior rating, which is the average of the ratings for the remaining five areas: relationship with patients, relationship with staff, reliability, responsibility, and emotional stability. For the purpose of this study, only the CCR was used to evaluate the utility of the PCX in classifying students' performances on the examination as satisfactory or unsatisfactory. The CCRs are often based on the ratings of one supervisor or, when available, on the averages of two supervisors' ratings. Because of the unavailability at the residency level of standardized and objective clinical-performance-evaluation data, the residency supervisors' ratings, although not the ultimate criterion for validating the PCX,[134] are presently the closest approximation to it and the only available evaluation of residents' clinical performances. For the class of 1987, the CCRs ranged from 4.9 to 9.9, with a mean of 7.5 and a standard deviation of 1.1; for the class of 1988 they ranged from 4.2 to 10.0, with a mean of 7.5 and a standard deviation of 1.4; and for the class of 1990, they ranged from 4.0 to 10.0, with a mean of 7.2 and a standard deviation of 1.2.

Because the students' CCRs were a function of the students' different residency programs and supervisors, and because none of the ratings obtained was found to be below average or unsatisfactory, a norm-referenced cutoff rating was used in this study to classify students as having a high residency performance rating (above the cutoff) or a low residency performance rating (below the cutoff) relative to their classmates. The cutoff was set at the class mean rating minus one standard deviation, resulting in a cutoff rating of 6.3 for the class of 1987, 6.1 for the class of 1988, and 6.1 for the class of 1990. Although on a scale from 1 (unsatisfactory) to 10 (outstanding) the ratings of 6.3 and 6.1 are equivalent to an average, or satisfactory, performance, these ratings may be considered low when compared across the three classes' rating distributions. It was found that the ranges of residency supervisors' ratings obtained here are representative of and similar to those found in other studies.[69,134,184] These results suggest that supervisors are reluctant to give very low ratings and that an assigned low or average (i.e., satisfactory) performance of a resident may reflect a relatively inferior performance.

Method of Analysis

Based on the PCX scores and the supervisors' rating cutoff scores, a 2×2 contingency table was set to determine how many of those students who received high or low supervisors' ratings in their first year of residency had performed satisfactorily or unsatisfactorily respectively on the PCX. It was expected that the students who received high ratings would have performed satisfactorily on the PCX and those who received low ratings would have performed unsatisfactorily on the PCX. The *sensitivity* of the PCX is then defined as the percentage of students who received high ratings in residency and had been identified correctly as satisfactory by the PCX. The *specificity* of the PCX is the percentage of students who received low ratings in residency and had been correctly identified as unsatisfactory by the PCX. We also calculated the rates of *false negatives* (the percentage of students receiving a high ratings in residency who had been incorrectly identified by the PCX as unsatisfactory) and *false positives* (the percentage of students receiving low ratings in residency who had been incorrectly identified by the PCX as satisfactory). Finally, the *predictive values* of the PCX were assessed by determining the probabilities that students classified as satisfactory or unsatisfactory on the PCX would receive high or low performance ratings in residency, respectively.

RESULTS

Using the PCX cutoff scores, we found that for the PCX of 1987, 40 of the 60 students who performed satisfactorily on the PCX (67%) and two of the six students who performed unsatisfactorily (33%) had supervisors' ratings on file. Similar results were obtained for the PCXs of 1988 and 1990; for the PCX of 1988, 41 of the 59 satisfactory students (69%) and six of the nine unsatisfactory students (55%) had supervisors' ratings on file; and for the PCX of 1990, 36 of the 51 satisfactory students (88%) and nine of the 14 unsatisfactory students (60%) had supervisors' ratings on file. Overall, for the classes of 1987, 1988, and 1990, there were 42, 46, and 45 students, respectively, or a total of 133 students, who had both PCX scores and supervisors' ratings on file. Most of the missing residency data were due to students' not giving permission for follow-up rather than to the supervisors' not responding. This study, like others (see Verhulst and Distlehorst, chapter 12), showed that the missing residency data were much greater among students who performed unsatisfactorily on the PCX or had poor academic performances in school than among those who performed satisfactorily on the PCX or had good academic performances in school.[160,184] The rates of missing data for those who performed satisfactorily on the PCXs of 1987,1988, and 1990 were 33%, 31% and 12%, respectively, while the corresponding rates of missing data for those performing unsatisfactorily were 67%, 45%, and 40%.

To describe the PCX overall test characteristics, results from the PCXs of 1987,1988, and 1990 were summarized in a 2×2 contingency table. Table 8.1 lists the frequencies of those students who had satisfactory or unsatisfactory performances on the PCX and received high or low supervisors' ratings, respectively, in their first year of residency. Based on these frequencies, we calculated the sensitivity and specificity

Table 8.1 Frequency Table of Numbers of Students Classified as Satisfactory (Sat.) or Unsatisfactory (Un.) on the Postclerkship Examination (PCX) and as Receiving High or Low Supervisors' Ratings in The First Year of Residency, Classes of 1987, 1988, and 1990, Southern Illinois University School of Medicine

	No. with High Rating	No. with Low Rating	Total
No. Sat.	103	14	117
No. Un.	10	6	16
TOTAL	113	20	133

PCX sensitivity: 103/113 = 91%.
PCX specificity: 6/20 = 30%.
PCX false–positive rate: 14/20 = 70%.
PCX false–negative rate: 10/113 = 9%.

of the PCXs, as well as the rates of false positives and false negatives, and the PCX predictive values.

The PCX was found to be very sensitive, in that for the three classes of students it correctly identified 91% (103 of 113) of those students who later received high ratings in the first year of residency. On the other hand, its specificity was much lower, in that it correctly identified only 30% (6 of 20) of the students who subsequently received low ratings in the first year of residency. Consequently, while there was a low false-negative error rate of 9% (10 of 113 students), the false-positive error rate was 70% (14 of 20 students). The PCX's predictive values suggest that while the test was accurate 88% of the time when predicting students who would obtain high ratings in the first year of residency (103 of 117 students), it was accurate only 38% of the time when predicting those students who would receive low ratings (6 of 16 students). Given the large proportion of missing residency performance data among students failing the PCX (40 to 67%), and given that students who did not give residency follow-up permission scored significantly lower on the PCX than those who did (see Verhulst and Distlehorst, chapter 12), the estimates of the PCX's sensitivity and specificity, of the rates of false positives and false negatives, and of the predictive values may be conservative. For example, if the residency data had been available for all students who failed the PCX and for those who did not give residency follow-up permission, the PCX's specificity might well have been higher and its sensitivity lower.

DISCUSSIONS AND CONCLUSIONS

The purpose of this study was to determine whether senior students' satisfactory or unsatisfactory performances on the standardized-patient-based postclerkship examination were predictive of their performance ratings in the first year of residency. Overall, the PCX was found to be more sensitive than specific, in that it identified more correctly those students who subsequently received high ratings in their residencies than those who received low ratings. Regarding the PCX's predictive value, it was found that while a great majority of those students who performed satisfactorily on the PCX could be predicted to receive high supervisors' ratings, only one-third of those who performed unsatisfactorily could be predicted to receive low supervisors' ratings. With its capability of identifying correctly students who will perform well in the first year of residency, the PCX can be a useful evaluation instrument to assess fourth-year medical students' readiness for promotion to residency. Given the moderate correlations of .45, .42, and .40 found between the students' PCX scores and their clerkship ratings, scores on the National Board of Medical Examiners Part I examination, and scores on the Part II examination, respectively,[191,192] it is important to determine next whether the PCX, when used in conjunction with these data, would improve the prediction of students' performances in residency.

To further assess the strengths and weaknesses of using students' performances on the PCX to predict their first-year residency performance ratings, we reviewed the comments that the supervisors provided to complement their ratings of the residents, so that we could uncover the reasons underlying those ratings. Of the 103 students who achieved satisfactory performances on the PCX and high supervisors' ratings, 98 (95%) had written comments from the supervisors. A great majority of these students (96%) received either satisfactory to excellent comments or no comments that were specific to their cognitive performances. A review of the supervisors' comments about those students who were correctly identified as receiving low supervisors' ratings further supported the utility of the PCX in identifying not only students' readiness but also their nonreadiness for residency. For example, the supervisors' comments available for five of the six students who performed unsatisfactorily on the PCX and had low supervisors' ratings showed that the low ratings were due to the residents' "weakness in general fund of knowledge," "differential diagnoses somewhat limited," or "inabilities to organize and interpret." Overall, the supervisors' comments for most of these residents were found to be consistent with their ratings.

Review of the supervisors' comments about those residents whose PCX scores were classified as false negative or false positive showed that for these residents the supervisors' comments were not always consistent with their ratings. For example, from the available comments for eight of the ten residents, whose PCX scores were classified as false negative, six comments referred to the resident's poor cognitive performances, such as "not as prepared for residency as other housestaff," or "relative weakness in thoroughness and organization." These comments suggest that the PCX did correctly identify the majority of these students as weak in their clinical performances and that even though their weaknesses were mentioned in the supervisors' comments, they were not reflected in the supervisors' ratings. Based on these data, it seems that most of the false negatives resulted from the inconsistencies found between the supervisors' ratings and their comments. These inconsistencies could result from the averaging of two divergent supervisors' ratings, and while the average rating may be above the cutoff, the unsatisfactory comments of one of the supervisors may still reflect the resident's performance.

Of the 14 students whose PCX scores were classified as false positive, only 6 (43%) were found to be correctly classified in that their low performance ratings matched their supervisors' comments. For the other eight students (57%), the supervisors' comments indicated that several reasons other than poor cognitive performance accounted for the low ratings. For example, three comments did not directly indicate the residents' poor performances except that the residents continued to improve in their performances, two comments indicated that the residents performed satisfactorily in the cognitive area but not in the noncognitive one, and three comments referred to the residents' unsatisfactory performances due to their preoccupations with changing their medical specialties.

In conclusion, by using the first-year residency supervisors' ratings as an indicator of students' postgraduate performances, we have shown that performance on the standardized-patient-based PCX is a relatively good indicator of both students' readiness and their nonreadiness for residency. Analyses of the supervisors' comments and ratings further supported the value of the PCX as a promising predictor, since they showed that most of the misclassifications could have been due more to the problems associated with the supervisors' ratings than with the PCX's inability to detect students' cognitive or clinical performance deficiencies.

CHAPTER NINE

Relationships of Interns' Performances to Their Self-Assessments of Their Preparedness for Internship and to Their Academic Performances in Medical School

Ruth-Marie E. Fincher, M.D., Lloyd A. Lewis, Ph.D., and Terrence T. Kuske, M.D.

There is no debate that successful completion of undergraduate medical school training is essential preparation for entry into a postgraduate residency training program. Therefore, it seems logical that undergraduate performance should be predictive of postgraduate performance. However, identifying which components of undergraduate medical education promote or predict performance during and after postgraduate training has been difficult. There are conflicting reports regarding what, if any, academic or personal characteristics correlate with subsequent performance. Undoubtedly this is due to the multivariate nature of the factors influencing postgraduate performance. Among these factors are student ability, the relevance of a specific medical school curriculum to any given specialty, difficulty in measuring clinical skills validly and reliably, and the variability of skills needed by residents in different postgraduate education programs. It is likely that medical school performance correlates better with performance in the intern year than with performance later in residency or in practice because the residency program itself may have more influence on later performance than does the medical school program.

Price and colleagues[144] concluded that medical school performance does not predict later professional performance, and Kron and colleagues[98] asserted that "no objective or subjective selection factor predicted the level of residency performance of those who completed the program." Neither of these studies attempted to predict performance in postgraduate year one (PGY-1) (the internship year). Wingard and Williamson,[202] however, found "little or no correlation between grades and career performance; grades did not correlate with immediate postgraduate performance." In contrast, Kegel-Flom[90] found that medical school grades and faculty ratings in the clinical years did predict intern performances. In concert with this conclusion, Veloski and colleagues[186] found that substantial numbers of good and poor performances in the PGY-1 year can be predicted on the basis of information available to medical school faculty. In 1987, Gunzburger and colleagues[60] concluded that intern performance as assessed by program directors can be predicted from scores on the National Board of Medical Examiners (NBME) Part II examination and clerkship grades. Studying a cohort of internal medicine residents in one residency program, Curry and colleagues[28] concluded that the NBME Part I scores, faculty evaluations, and academic distinction were the strongest predictors of performance; academic distinction was the single strongest predictor. Studying surgery residents' performances in one program, Erlandson and colleagues[35] found that medical school honors constituted a variable that correlated with performance on the American Board of Surgery In Training Examination, but found no correlation between the honors variables (preclinical and clinical core honors) and factor indices of knowledge and personal skill. A recent study by Loftus and colleagues[110] concluded that medical school ranking, as assessed by any of three ranking systems, showed a modest correlation with residency performance. The ranking systems involved computation of an index based on the dean's letter, a norm-referenced system, and a criterion-based system.

While students are frequently asked to evaluate the housestaff and attending physicians with whom they work, they are not often asked to assess their own performances. This is unfortunate, because self-assessment and consequent recognition of one's educational needs are important for self-motivated, continuing medical education.[64] Nonetheless, there are several studies analyzing students' self-evaluations. Arnold and colleagues[9] have shown that students' self-evaluations and faculty's evaluations of the students both rose throughout the course of medical school training, but the strength of the correlation between the two kinds of evaluations decreased as the year progressed. In contrast, Peters and Schimpfhauser[138] found that students tended to rate themselves higher than the faculty rated them. Studying second-year students self-, peer, and faculty evaluations, Calhoun and colleagues[21] reported that the ratings on the self- and peer evaluations were similar, but differed significantly from the ratings on the faculty evaluations. Others[124] have found that students tend to rate themselves about the same as or lower than the faculty do.

Both because of the importance of self-assessment in continuing education and as a measure in educational outcomes research, we at the Medical College of Georgia (MCG) have begun a process of self- and program director evaluation for students during the intern year. The student evaluation questionnaire used at MCG was similar to those used in the self-assessment studies in the literature, but differs slightly in that it was actually an assessment of the quality of academic preparation for the intern year.

Our initial motivation for collecting data from students regarding their self-evaluations of preparedness for internship and from internship program directors regarding students' performances as interns was as an assessment of our medical school curriculum as preparation for postgraduate training. In addition, we had the opportunity to analyze the relationship between our students' medical school and internship performances, and the correlation between students' self-assessments of preparedness for internship and their program directors' evaluations of their performances. In this study, we assessed the relationship between the undergraduate performances of the 1990 and 1991 graduating classes of the MCG School of Medicine and the performances of this cohort of students in the internship year. This study addressed three research questions: (1) Does cumulative medical school grade-point average (GPA) predict program directors' assessment (ranking) of overall performance? (2) Does medical school academic performance predict performances in specific areas of competency as assessed by program directors? (3) Do students' self-assessments of preparedness for internship correlate with the program director's evaluations of those same areas of competency?

METHOD

We developed a questionnaire to assess interns' overall competency and their competencies in nine specific areas. The instrument was based on ones previously developed and used by other medical schools to evaluate their former students during the internship year. This instrument was sent to the 1990 and 1991 graduates of the MCG School of Medicine who were interns and who consented to participate in the study; it was also sent to the directors of the interns' programs. Specifically, in January 1991 we sent questionnaires to the 1990 graduates and to their program directors, and in January 1992 the questionnaires were sent to the 1991 graduates and their program directors. We also sent forms to all the interns requesting that they allow their program directors to release their (interns') evaluations to us; we gave the program directors the signed forms that were returned to us.

The response options on the questionnaire were on a five-point Likert scale that ranged from 1, unsatisfactory, to 5, outstanding. Except for two questions, the questionnaires sent to the interns and their program directors were identical. The program directors, but not the interns, were asked to evaluate each intern's initiative and willingness to research problems in the literature. The directors were also asked to rank each intern as being in the top, middle, or lower third of his or her group of interns. Each intern was asked to rank himself or herself as being in the top, middle, or lower third of the group in terms of his or her degree of preparation to begin the internship.

A total of 138 (80%) of the 173 graduates of the class of 1990 and 145 (83%) of the 174 1991 graduates consented to have the program directors release their evaluations to us. For the class of 1990, this included 76% of the students in the top third of the class, 83% in the middle third, and 41% in the bottom third. For the class of 1991, it included 79% of those in the upper third, 54% in the middle third, and 68% in the bottom third. The program directors' response rates were 83% (114 completed ratings) for the class of 1990 and 72% (104 completed ratings) for the class of 1991. This represents 66% of the total class of 1990 and 60% of the class of 1991. One hundred thirty-three (38%) of the students completed the self-assessment questionnaire. Only one mailing was sent.

All correlations were estimated using Pearson correlation coefficients. Associations between medical school class rankings and program directors' rankings were examined using cross tabulations. Significance was tested using a chi-square test. A contingency coefficient was used to assess the magnitude of association between these two types of rankings. A multivariate analysis of variance was used to test for differences between means of specific competencies between the classes of 1990 and 1991. The significance level was set at alpha $< .05$.

Table 9.1 Numbers of Interns Ranked in The Top, Middle, and Bottom Thirds of (1) Their Medical School Classes (by Academic Performance), and (2) Their Internship Groups (by Overall Performance), Medical College of Georgia Classes of 1990 and 1991*

	Internship Rank			
Medical School Rank	**No. in Top Third**	**No. in Middle Third**	**No. in Bottom Third**	**Total**
No. in top third	57	20	2	79
No. in middle third	50	31	4	85
No. in bottom third	20	21	13	54
TOTAL	127	72	19	218

$\chi^2 = 28.7$; df = 4; $p = .0001$.
Contingency coefficient = .34
*The class rankings were based on the student's overall grade-point averages; the internship rankings were made by the program directors.

RESULTS

One hundred seven (49%) of the students in the two classes selected postgraduate training in one of the primary care specialties of internal medicine, family medicine, or pediatrics. The remaining 110 (51%) chose non-primary-care specialties. One hundred sixteen (54%) of the graduates were interns in university-based training programs and 100 (46%) were in community programs at the time the study was done. There was no significant relationship between the program directors' ratings of interns in the top, middle, and bottom third of their groups and whether the students were in the university or the community programs. Students who chose residency training in university programs had significantly higher medical school GPAs than did those who chose community programs.

The correlation between cumulative and clinical GPAs was .91. Therefore only the cumulative GPA was used for further analysis. Cross-tabulations of medical school GPA rankings with the program directors' rankings of students by thirds in the intern training program are shown in Table 9.1. The contingency coefficient for cumulative rankings of medical school GPAs with program directors' rankings by thirds is .34, significant at $p < .0001$; the maximum contingency for a 3×3 table is .82.

Each student's cumulative medical school GPA was correlated with program directors' ratings of competencies in specific areas. The com-

Table 9.2 Mean Scores in Specific Competency Areas (1) Interns' Self-assessments of Preparedness for Internship, and (2) Program Directors' Assessments of Interns' Performances, Medical College of Georgia, Classes of 1990 and 1991*

Area of Competency	Mean Score from Program Director	Mean Score from Self-Assessment
Fund of basic science and clinical knowledge	3.7	3.7
Ability to take a thorough and relevant history	3.9	3.9
Ability to perform an appropriate physical examination	3.9	3.8
Ability to order and interpret laboratory tests relevant to the problem confronted	3.8	3.5
Ability to arrive at an appropriate differential diagnosis	3.8	3.5
Ability to propose and implement appropriate management for all patients	3.8	3.5
Ability to provide continuing and extended care for patients	3.9	3.4
Ability to perform manual skills as needed	3.9	4.0
Demonstrates initiative by expressing an interest in continued willingness to research problems in the literature, etc.	4.3	—
Relates well to patients, support staff, colleagues, attending physicians, etc.	4.3	4.0
Overall ability as a houseofficer	3.9	4.0

*Assessments were made on a Likert scale, from 1, unsatisfactory, to 5, outstanding. There were 114 program directors' assessments of the performances of interns who had been in the MCG's class of 1990. For the class of 1991, there were 104 program directors' assessments and 70 interns' self-assessments.

petencies shown in Table 9.2 were significantly correlated with the student's GPA. Correlation coefficients ranged from .28 to .51; since most ratings ranged from 3 to 5 on the 1 to 5 rating scale, the correlation coefficients may have been underestimated. Program directors' assessments and interns' self-assessments in each of the nine areas of competency are shown in Table 9.2.

Program directors' evaluations shown for 1990 and 1991 were combined because there was no significant difference between the two years. Because of an error in the response options of the 1990 questionnaire, data are shown only for the class of 1991 for self-assessment, except for the ranking of preparedness. The program directors' mean assessment of the interns was slightly higher than the interns' mean self-assessment in most areas of competency. The correlation between mean self-ratings and mean program directors' ratings of specific competencies equals .58 with 8 degrees of freedom. Because of the small number, this is not statistically significant at the .05 level. The correlation would have to have been .63 to have been statistically significant. Lack of statistical significance should not overshadow the magnitude of the relationship.

Program directors ranked one hundred twenty-six (58%) of the students in the upper third of their intern groups, 72 (33%) in the middle third, and 20 (9.2%) in the lower third. Students' self-ratings of their preparedness for internship placed 77 (58%) in the upper third, 54 (41%) in the middle third, and two (1%) in the lower third. Although 25% of the students who consented to have their program directors release information about their internship performances were ranked in the lower third of the class, only 9.2% were ranked in the lower third regarding their actual performances.

DISCUSSION

Although 82% of the students in both classes consented to have information released by their program directors, we also analyzed whether the consenting and nonconsenting groups were similar. For each class, higher percentages of students in the upper and middle thirds than in the lower third consented. However, when the two classes were combined, more than half of the lower third also consented. As MCG students are not informed of their numerical class rankings, their self-assessments regarding preparation for internship are based solely on their perceptions of performance. There was no significant difference in correlations between Medical College Admission Test (MCAT) scores and cumulative medical school GPAs for the consenting versus the nonconsenting students.

Our data suggest that medical school academic performance as estimated by the cumulative medical school GPA predicts both overall performance and specific competencies as assessed by the program director for the internship year. Presumably because of the close correlation (.91), this would be true for the clinical medical school GPA as well. As this study involved only performance in the intern year and not performance at the more advanced levels of training or in practice, we cannot test our suggestion that medical school performance correlates most closely with internship performance. Further investigation of these and other classes as they reach the end of training is needed to address that question. However, it is plausible that one reason several previous studies[98,144,202] have found no correlation between medical school and subsequent performances is that their outcome measures were obtained at the end of residency or during practice. Similarly, this may explain why several other studies[60,90,186] showed predictive relationships between medical school and internship performances. The nature of the relationship between medical school performance and performance in practice remains unclear, but undoubtedly involves characteristics of both the medical school and the residency. The present study examined only the predictive relationship of medical school academic performance, as estimated by the medical school GPA, with internship performance, as assessed by the program director's evaluation.

Program directors rated our graduates highly in all areas of competence, with no significant difference between the years. This finding suggests that the performances of graduates are similar from year to year. As the undergraduate curricula were similar for the two classes and the demographic characteristics of the classes were similar, the similarity in ratings was anticipated. Interestingly, at least half of the students who ranked in the middle third and more than a third of those in the bottom third of their graduating classes were ranked by their program directors in the top thirds of their intern groups.

The finding that our students generally gave themselves lower ratings than their program directors did is consistent with findings of other studies of self-assessment.[9,14] While the correlation between self- and program-director assessment did not reach statistical significance, we believe this relationship is important, because more experience in self-assessment during training might improve the accuracy of self-assessment, which would be valuable for assessment of one's performance in practice.

There is no dispute that medical school education provides the foundation for postgraduate training. However, more study is needed to identify which components of medical school education and which personal characteristics promote laudatory performances during and after postgraduate training.

CHAPTER TEN

Validity of NBME Part I and Part II Scores for Selection of Residents in Orthopaedic Surgery, Dermatology, and Preventive Medicine

Susan M. Case, Ph.D., and David B. Swanson, Ph.D.

In trying to select the best residents from large numbers of applicants, program directors face a challenging task. They commonly use scores from the National Board of Medical Examiners (NBME) Part I and Part II examinations as one source of information about applicants.[119,193,194] Use of NBME scores, in effect, "levels the playing field," providing students at less prestigious schools with the opportunity to be considered for entry into highly selective training programs. In addition, other measures, such as medical school grades and dean's letters, have problems with comparability and interpretability.[193] However, use of NBME scores for selection of residents has been criticized because neither the Part I nor the Part II examinations were developed for this purpose; in addition, the time lag between taking the examinations (particularly Part I) and residency training is large, and the content (especially of Part I) seems only indirectly related to the knowledge required in residency.[190] While much of this debate has been philosophical (and polemical), these criticisms do raise an important empirical issue concerning the relationship between NBME scores and performances in residency: How accurately do NBME scores predict criterion measures of success in residency training? Despite widespread use of NBME scores for the selection of residents, there is little published information relating NBME scores to actual performances in residency training. Investigations using in-training examinations as criterion measures have produced inconsistent results, perhaps because these studies have generally been based on small sample sizes, including residents from single programs.[24,171,196] Other studies have shown consistently positive but weak relationships, using faculty ratings of resident performances as criterion measures[31,41,89,115,184,187,200,206]; these results may simply reflect psychometric weaknesses commonly associated with ratings (e.g., poor interrater reliability, halo effects, bias). Questions raised by the American Board of Orthopaedic Surgery regarding the utility of NBME Part I scores for the selection of residents prompted a series of studies by the first author (SMC). In contradistinction to research that has used in-training examination scores or faculty ratings as indicators of success in residency, this work used performance on the orthopaedic specialty examination for board certification as the criterion measure. Because the results showed an unexpectedly high predictive relationship, the study was replicated several times, and ultimately, two additional studies of other board examinations were conducted; the latter boards were believed to provide a contrast, particularly in terms of requisite knowledge, to orthopaedics. This article reports the results of the three studies, which relate performance on NBME Part I and Part II examinations to scores on the 1991 certification examinations of the American Board of Orthopaedic Surgery (ABOS), the American Board of Dermatology (ABD), and the American Board of Preventive Medicine (ABPM). The article is organized into five sections. The first describes the NBME scores used in the studies. The following three sections present the methods, results, and discussions for the three individual studies. The final section discusses the conclusions that follow after analyzing the three studies jointly.

NBME SCORES USED IN THE STUDIES

The scores used in the three studies reported here are based on NBME Part I and Part II scores, statistically equated across all administrations of a given Part examination. In general, the scores fall between 200 and 800, and, depending upon the test administration, the mean and standard deviation are approximately 500 and 100, respectively, for examinees sitting for the NBME Part examinations for the first time. Using procedures discussed below, Part I and Part II scores were retrieved for examinees taking the 1991 certifying examinations of the three specialty boards. For the examinees who took Part I or Part II more than once, the last score they received was used in analyses, because this score would typically be the score sent to residency program directors. Scores were unavailable for pre-1979 test administrations. The amounts of missing data varied across the specialty board examinations, and the extent to which each sample differed from the associated examinee population taking the specialty board examination is addressed in presentation of the individual studies.

STUDY 1: ORTHOPAEDIC SURGERY

Method

Subjects

A total of 870 examinees took the ABOS written certifying examination in 1991; the study sample included 656 examinees (75%), who were identified in the NBME database via social security numbers. NBME Part I scores were found for 621 examinees, and NBME Part II scores were found for 623. The missing 25% of the examinee population included 88 (10%) graduates of foreign medical schools; the remainder were graduates of United States or Canadian schools who were not found in the database.

Instrumentation

The ABOS examination was administered in a single site under secure conditions. The six-hour examination included 277 multiple-choice questions (MCQs). The examination assessed the examinees' application of knowledge through the use of clinical vignettes combined with more than 150 radiographs, histosections, or other pictorial material that required the examinees to interpret the information and formulate a diagnosis or a management plan. The scores used in this study are expressed on a percentage-correct scale. Test reliability (coefficient alpha) was .92.

Results and Discussion

Characteristics of the Sample

The representativeness of the study sample was investigated by comparing the performances on the 1991 ABOS examination of the sample (i.e., those for whom NBME scores were available) and the total group (all those who took the 1991 ABOS examination). The study sample performed somewhat better overall (mean, 78; SD, 6.4) than the total group (mean, 76; SD, 8.4), partially reflecting the poorer performance of graduates of foreign medical schools (mean, 64; SD, 9.1), who were ineligible for NBME examinations. Lower performance was also seen in the repeater candidates (mean, 66; SD, 8.2), who were underrepresented in the study sample (13% of the sample and 22% of the total group). The study sample, thus, was a somewhat more able and homogeneous group than the total group. The restriction in range in the study sample results in a conservative (attenuated) estimate of the strength of the relationship between NBME and specialty board scores.

Performance on NBME Examinations

The overall average mean scores for the study sample were 518 (SD = 99) on NBME Part I and 483 (SD = 107) on NBME Part II. Of particular interest is the pattern of subscore means, which were relatively high for anatomy (537) on Part I and surgery (524) on Part II; the lowest mean scores were on behavioral sciences (496) for Part I and psychiatry (470) for Part II. This pattern seems consistent with content emphases in orthopaedic surgery.

Correlations Between Scores

Statistically significant relationships were found between scores on the ABOS examination and all NBME Part examinations. As shown in Table 10.1, scores on the ABOS examination had observed correlations of .59 with NBME Part I and .64 with Part II. The strongest correlations with Part I subtests were with anatomy (.54) and physiology (.54), followed by pharmacology (.48) and pathology (.48); the weakest correlation was with behavioral sciences (.38). The strongest correlations with Part II subtests were with surgery (.61), medicine (.58), and pediatrics (.55), while the weakest relationships were with psychiatry (.46) and preventive medicine and public health (PMPH) (.49). The pattern of correlations also seems consistent with expectations based on the content of the measures.

Prediction of ABOS Scores

Regression analyses were performed using ABOS scores as the dependent (criterion) variable and various combinations of NBME scores as the independent (predictor) variables. The most accurate prediction of ABOS scores was obtained by using the combination of all NBME Part I and Part II subscores (adjusted multiple correlation of .68); however, this prediction was only slightly more accurate than using Part II subscores alone (.66), total scores from both Parts (.65), or the NBME Part II total score alone (.64). Using Part I total scores alone (.59) and Part I subscores alone (.60) produced slightly less accurate predictions of ABOS scores.

Table 10.1 Correlations between Specialty Board Certification Examination Scores and National Board of Medical Examiners (NBME) Examination Scores

NBME Score	American Board of Orthopaedic Surgery	American Board of Dermatology		American Board of Preventive Medicine
		Non-PIX*	PIX*	
Part I total	59	49	42	63
Anatomy	54	34	34	44
Physiology	54	43	35	66
Biochemistry	46	49	38	48
Pathology	48	42	38	44
Microbiology	46	44	33	54
Pharmacology	48	40	32	46
Behavioral Sciences	38	25	24	49
Sample size	621	214	214	133
Part II total	64	48	51	68
Medicine	58	47	51	57
Surgery	61	44	53	52
Obstetrics–gynecology	51	38	44	39
PMPH†	49	30	30	64
Pediatrics	55	42	41	45
Psychiatry	46	38	34	55
Sample size	623	204	204	151

*PIX = pictorial examination.
†Preventive medicine and public health.

Failure Rates on the ABOS Examination

A total of 83 (13%) of the 656 examinees in the study sample failed the ABOS examination. Figure 10.1 shows the proportion of those who failed the ABOS examination as a function of performance on the Part I and II examinations. A strong relationship was present between performance on NBME examinations and ABOS pass–fail results. For example, for NBME Part I, 38% of those scoring below 400 failed the ABOS examination, while only 1.6% of those scoring above 600 failed; thus the risk for failing is more than 20 times as great in the lowest-scoring group. A similar pattern was observed for NBME Part II.

STUDY 2: DERMATOLOGY

Method

Subjects

The study sample included 219 (73%) of the 302 examinees who took the certification examination of the ABD in 1991; they were identified in the NBME database via examinee names; social security num-

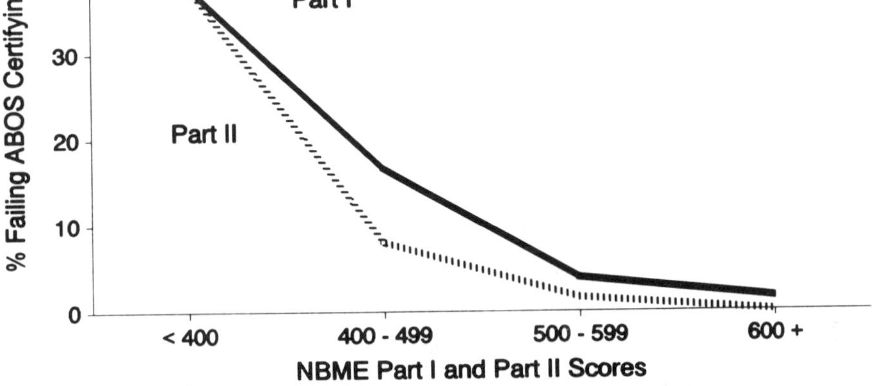

Figure 10.1 Relationship Between ABOS Failure Rates and NBME Performance.

bers were not available. NBME scores were obtained for 214 examinees on NBME Part I and 204 examinees on NBME Part II. The missing 27% of the examinee population include 12 graduates of foreign medical schools (4%); the remainder were U.S. or Canadian graduates for whom NBME scores were unavailable.

Instrumentation

The ABD examination was administered in a single site under secure conditions. It included two major components. The first was a non-pictorial examination (termed non-PIX hereafter) with approximately 250 MCQs; the items focused primarily on recall of basic science information, recognition of symptoms associated with specific diagnoses, interpretation of laboratory data, and identification of appropriate treatments for various diagnoses. The second examination was a pictorial examination (termed PIX hereafter) with approximately 350 items, most of which required the examinees to identify disorders depicted on slides that were shown during test administration. Each component of the ABD examination is scored separately; the examinees may pass individual components, but must eventually pass both in order to be certified. Test reliabilities were .92 and .90 for the non-PIX and PIX components, respectively.

Results and Discussion

Characteristics of the Sample

The representativeness of the study sample was investigated by comparing the certifying examination performance of the sample with that of the total group. Means for the non-PIX component were 485 (SD = 115) for the sample and 477 (SD = 124) for the total group. Means for the PIX component were 495 (SD = 92) for the sample and 489 (SD = 96) for the total group. Thus, the groups were quite similar.

Performance on NBME Examinations

The mean performance scores for the study sample on Parts I and II were 506 and 493, respectively. The highest subscore means were on pharmacology (518) for Part I and medicine (499) for Part II.

Correlations Between Scores

As shown in Table 2, statistically significant relationships were found between all scores on the ABD and NBME examinations. NBME Part

I total scores were more highly related to the non-PIX examination scores (r = .49) than to the PIX examination scores (r = .42); the reverse was true of NBME Part II (r's = .48 for non-PIX and .51 for PIX). The correlations between NBME Part I subtest scores and the non-PIX examination scores ranged from .25 with behavioral sciences to .49 with biochemistry; correlations with the PIX examination scores ranged from .24 with behavioral sciences to .38 with pathology. The correlations between NBME Part II subtest scores and the ABD examination scores were highest for medicine and surgery; the weakest relationships were with psychiatry and PMPH. The pattern of correlations seems interpretable in terms of examination content: (1) relatively strong relationships between scores on the PIX examination and the disciplines of Parts I and II with a more visual focus (pathology and surgery); (2) relatively strong relationships with medicine and surgery for both ABD examinations; and (3) relatively weak relationships with behavioral sciences, psychiatry, and PMPH.

Prediction of ABD Scores

Regression analyses indicated that NBME Part I and NBME Part II were almost equally accurate in predicting performance on the non-PIX examination (adjusted multiple correlations of .49 and .48, respectively); however, NBME Part II was a better predictor of performance on the PIX examination than Part I (adjusted multiple correlations of .51 and .42, respectively). As in the ABOS study, use of NBME subscores as predictors was only slightly more accurate, at best, than use of NBME total scores alone. The primary distinction between these results and those using ABOS data was the relatively weak predictive value of NBME Part I in predicting PIX scores.

Failure Rates on the ABD Examination

A total of 39 (18%) of the 219 examinees in the study sample failed one or both components of the ABD examination. Figure 2 shows the percentage of examinees failing the ABD examination as a function of performance on the NBME Part I and Part II examinations. As in the ABOS study, there was a strong relationship between performance on the NBME examinations and ABD pass–fail results. For Part I, 56% of those scoring below 400 failed the ABD examination, while none of those scoring above 600 failed. For Part II, the analogous percentages were 51% and 3%, respectively.

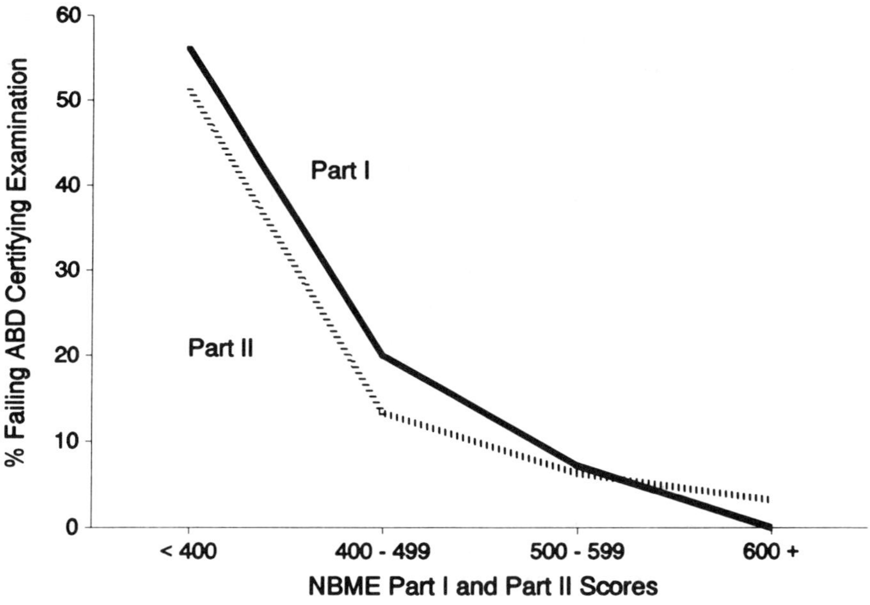

Figure 10.2 Relationship Between ABD Failure Rates and NBME Performance.

STUDY 3: PREVENTIVE MEDICINE

Method

Subjects

Of the 427 candidates sitting for the ABPM certifying examination in 1991, 169 (40%) were identified in the NBME database by matching the names and year of medical school graduation; social security numbers were not available. Part I scores were obtained for 133 examinees; Part II scores were located for 151 examinees. The missing 60% of the examinee population included 107 (25%) graduates of foreign medical schools. The remaining 187 (35%) missing examinees were United States or Canadian graduates for whom NBME scores were unavailable; 119 (28%) had graduated from medical school before 1979, the first year included in the NBME database. Thus, the large number of examinees missing from this study sample reflects, in part, later career entry of experienced physicians into preventive medicine, as well as a larger proportion of graduates of foreign medical schools than in the other studies.

Instrumentation

The ABPM examination was administered in a single site under secure conditions. To be certified, examinees must pass both a 250-item Core examination and one of three specialty examinations (not discussed in this paper). Four hours were allotted for the Core examination; it covered topics in environmental medicine, biostatistics, epidemiology, clinical prevention, and behavioral medicine. The scores used in the study are expressed on a percentage-correct scale. Test reliability (coefficient alpha) was .94.

Results and Discussion

Characteristics of the Sample

The representativeness of the study sample was investigated by comparing the scores of the study sample with those of the total group. The sample performed better overall (mean, 75; SD, 7.8) than the total group (mean, 68; SD, 11.1), reflecting the somewhat lower performances of older candidates and graduates of foreign schools. Because the study sample was more able and homogeneous than the total group, observed relationships with NBME performance may be somewhat attenuated.

Performance on NBME Examinations

The pattern of subtest means was almost the reverse of the pattern for the ABOS: highest for behavioral sciences, PMPH, and psychiatry and lowest for anatomy and surgery. Given the knowledge and skills emphasized in preventive medicine training and in the ABPM examination, relatively strong performance in quantitative, behavioral sciences, and, of course, PMPH areas seems quite natural.

Correlations Between Scores

As in the first two studies, statistically significant relationships were found between the ABPM examinations and all NBME scores. The ABPM Core examination score had observed correlations of .63 with Part I and .68 with Part II. ABPM scores were most strongly correlated with subscores in physiology (.65), microbiology (.54), behavioral sciences (.49), PMPH (.64), medicine (.57), and psychiatry (.55). This correlational pattern is distinctly different from those observed in the first two studies, yet also interpretable in terms of content relationships among the areas.

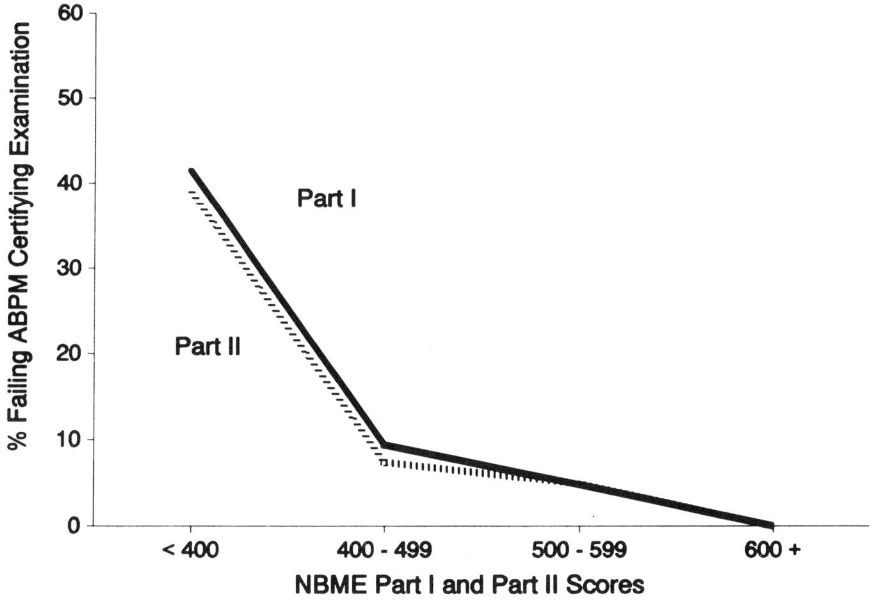

Figure 10.3 Relationship Between ABPM Failure Rates and NBME Performance.

Prediction of ABPM Scores

As with the ABOS and the ABD, regression analyses indicated that the NBME Part II total score provided a more accurate prediction of ABPM scores than did the NBME Part I total score (adjusted multiple correlations .68 versus .63). However, in contradistinction to the results for the ABOS and the ABD, the NBME Part I and Part II subscores provided more accurate predictions. Use of the combination of Part I and II subscores yielded an adjusted multiple correlation of .78. Use of the combination of NBME Part I and Part II total scores yielded an adjusted multiple correlation of .68, the same as Part II alone.

Failure Rates on the ABPM Examination

A total of 23 (14%) of the 169 examinees in the study sample failed one or both components of the ABPM examination. Figure 10.3 shows the percentage of examinees failing the ABPM examination as a function of performance on the NBME Part I and II examinations. Once again there were very strong relationships between performance on NBME examinations and ABPM pass–fail results: those performing poorly on NBME Part I and Part II had a substantially increased risk for failing the ABPM examination.

GENERAL DISCUSSION

The overall results were quite consistent and interpretable across studies. The patterns of high and low mean scores on NBME Part I and Part II subtests were generally related to the skills required in the specialty areas. This may reflect the examinees' preferences in specialty selection or the residency programs' preferences in resident selection. Similarly, correlations between specialty board performance and NBME Part I and Part II subscores tended to be higher for subtest areas more closely related to the specialty. In regression analyses, NBME Part I and Part II scores provided a good basis for predicting specialty board performance. NBME Part II scores generally provided a better basis for predicting specialty board performance than did Part I scores, probably reflecting both the greater similarity of the test material and the shorter time span between test administrations for Part II and specialty board examinations. Use of *both* Part I and Part II total scores markedly improved predictions of ABD Non-PIX, but not ABOS, ABPM, or ABD PIX performance. Use of subscores, rather than total scores, markedly improved the predictive accuracy of ABPM performance, although use of the Part II total score alone was at least as accurate as any combination of scores for the other boards. In all three studies, strong relationships were observed between specialty board pass–fail outcomes and Part I and Part II scores: examinees with Part I or Part II scores below 400 were at much greater risk for failing the specialty board certification examinations.

Thus, the three studies strongly support the common observation that those who have done well on examinations in the past continue to do well on examinations. This result, while mildly interesting, can be explored further by looking at three potential explanations. The first explanation, often voiced by critics of multiple-choice testing, is that examination performance is largely a reflection of test-taking skills, not knowledge. Because good test-taking skills and high test scores are a virtual necessity in order to gain entry to medical school, we do not find this argument particularly compelling; most examinees at this level have reasonably good test-taking skills. In addition, if this explanation were correct, the correlations between NBME scores and the specialty board scores should be very similar for all Part I and Part II subtests, and this was *not* the case in any of the three studies.

A second potential explanation for the strong observed relationships is that performances on both NBME and specialty board examinations indirectly reflect general ability, motivation, study skills, and other general traits that influence success in learning. Past achievement may be a good predictor of future achievement because of this indirect relationship. While there may be an element of truth in this explanation, it does not tell the whole story; the variation in the magnitudes of the correlations between specialty board performances and NBME subscores is too great.

The pattern of correlations suggests a third explanation: scores provide direct information about an examinee's knowledge in "job-related" subareas of interest. The correlations between NBME subscores and specialty board performances ranged from .25 to .66, and the pattern of correlations is interpretable in terms of overlap in examination content and the knowledge and skills required to practice the specialty. While little of the content covered by Part I is directly measured on the specialty board examinations, much of the content provides a framework for the knowledge assessed on the later examinations. For the ABOS, the relationships with anatomy and physiology plus those in medicine and surgery were relatively strong, while the relationships with behavioral sciences, psychiatry, and PMPH were relatively weak. For the ABD, the relationship between the PIX examination score and scores in disciplines with a major pictorial focus was notable. As with the ABOS, the relationships between ABD scores and performances on the behavioral sciences, psychiatry, and PMPH subtests were relatively weak; this pattern was in marked contrast to that for the ABPM, where the relationships were much stronger for these disciplines.

Despite the relatively strong and consistent results, there are several reasons why these results must be interpreted with caution. First, the investigation included only three specialty board examinations; even though the specialties studied are quite diverse, the results may not generalize to other specialties. Replication studies involving additional test administrations for the included specialty boards as well as additional specialties, are planned for the future. Second, the study included only a subset of examinees who took the specialty board examinations. For all three specialties, the study samples performed better than the total examinee groups on the specialty board examinations; this restriction of range should have the effect of, if anything, underestimating the magnitude of the relationships. Third, NBME Parts I and II have been replaced by USMLE Steps 1 and 2. While it is possible that correlations with individual subscores would differ, it is unlikely that the overall strengths of the relationships based on total scores would diminish, and it is the total scores that are available for USMLE examinations.

The last, and probably the most serious, limitation is the use of performance on specialty board examinations as a criterion measure: these written test scores clearly fall short of a "gold standard" for assessing clinical competence. However, such a gold standard probably does not exist, and the use of certification examination performance is a reasonable alternative. Specialty certification examination performance is of significant practical importance to program directors, because of links to the accreditation of training programs. Furthermore, these examinations are reliable, professionally developed measures of the cognitive components of clinical competence that are widely accepted and used by the medical community.

While we think that the results of these studies provide strong empirical support for the use of NBME Part I and Part II examinations in selection of residents, we do not endorse the use of these examination scores as a sole determinant of acceptance into residency programs. Many traits not measured by written tests are clearly important to success in residency training; these traits should also be considered in selection of residents. In addition, the relationship between NBME scores and specialty board performances is substantially less than perfect: some examinees with low NBME scores passed each of the specialty board examinations. At the same time, all three studies showed that NBME Part I and Part II scores predict performances on certification examinations taken many years later. Strong relationships were found between performance on NBME examinations and failure rates on specialty board examinations. NBME scores appear to provide an efficient and effective method for screening applicants before interviews, especially for programs that have many more applicants than positions.

CHAPTER ELEVEN

Lifelong Learning of Physicians: Contributions of Different Educational Phases to Practice Performance

Hans E. Renschler, Dr. Med., and
Ute Fuchs, Dr. Med. Habil.

Learning in medicine is directed toward achieving the best possible patient care. Physicians are subjected to different phases of teaching and training in the guise of preclinical, clinical, and postgraduate education. After the completion of formal training, they must update their knowledge and skills to keep up the quality of their performances. However, teaching does not equal learning, and learning does not equal competence or even performance, which is the measurable outcome of learning.[152] It is not known to what degree each phase of a physician's training contributes to his or her daily medical practice. But it is clear that some of the knowledge the physician has acquired in learning the basic and clinical sciences will become obsolete.

Knowledge learned in basic sciences that is not oriented to symptoms and diseases is not retained in a form that can be applied to solving clinical problems.[137] Skills must be acquired actively, are refined in the clinical setting,[56] and are related to the learner's most recent experience. Thus, knowledge acquired in earlier educational phases loses significance. The influence of medical school in providing a common knowledge base is limited in scope and is reversed by clinical practice.[57]

The quality of the daily work of doctors depends to a large extent on the opportunities for learning available to them and on the effectiveness of the reward systems in which they participate. Rich and coworkers concluded from their investigation of the effects of interventions that practice is subject to a variety of influences involving not only knowledge and the practice environment but also training, professional attitudes, and health beliefs.[155] Even though problem-based learning is considered to be best suited for professional updating in practice-based learning, it was not kept up by graduates of the McMaster University School of Medicine.[183]

If one concludes from these studies that the efficacy of undergraduate medical education is limited with regard to the practice of medicine, then a great amount of learning should occur during the postgraduate phases of training. However, there are no data evidencing the contributions of the individual phases of physicians' medical education to clinical performance. It would be difficult, if not impossible, to measure the contribution of each phase with common goals for all physicians, because of the differences in their ultimate individual tasks.

This pilot study was designed to find out how physicians perceived where and when they had acquired the competencies they used in their daily practices five years after the completion of their formal training. In Germany there is a uniform curriculum for medical education. It consists of two years of preclinical and three years of clinical education based mainly on lectures and demonstrations. The sixth year, a "practical year," is spent in a teaching hospital. A second practical phase of 18 months' duration, the "physician-in-practice year," was added in the autumn of 1988. (For more information about the German health care system, see the excellent description and evaluation by Iglehart.[79,80])

Self-ratings can give reliable and valid measurements of a variety of constructs.[92] We asked a group of physicians participating in a continuing medical education (CME) course to what degrees the knowledge and skills they had acquired in the different phases of their training had contributed to their daily medical practice. In this paper we report the results of that survey.

METHOD

We developed and revised a one-page questionnaire and handed it out in November, 1991 to the 330 physicians participating in a traditional CME seminar on emergency medicine. The participants were given a short explanation of the questions.

In addition to demographic data, the physicians were asked to provide information on certification and employment, and whether they participated in local workshops or study groups designed to improve the medical practices of the individual participants. They were asked to estimate what percentage each of seven phases of their medical education had contributed to their practices of medicine five years after the completion of their postgraduate training (the total of these percentages being 100%). The seven phases of medical education were preclinical, clinical, "practical year" (practice phase 1), "physician-in-practice year" (practice phase 2), specialty training or work as junior attendant physician, formal CME (lectures with discussion), and practice-based independent learning. We also provided a section for open-ended remarks. A standard statistical package was used to analyze the results.[132]

Of the 330 participants, 141 returned the completed questionnaire; 114 of these were suitable for evaluation (27 were excluded because they were incomplete or incorrectly filled out). The mean age of the respondents was 33.1 years (range 26–71), with a median year of licensure of 1986 (range 1945–1992); 18 (16%) of the respondents were certified as specialists; 84 (74%) were hospital-based (60 in a city, 11 in a rural area, and 13 in a university hospital); 44 (39%) participated regularly in local CME study groups or workshops.

RESULTS

The percentages of the contributions of the seven training phases to the physicians' medical practices, given as median and range (in parentheses), were as follows: 5% (0–30%) for preclinical education; 10% (0–60%) for clinical education; 15% (0–40%) for the practical year; 5% (0–70%) for practice phase 2; 20% (0–80%) for specialty training; 5% (0–30%) for formal CME; and 18% (0–90%) for independent learning. Medians are given because the frequency distribution of the data is not normal.

According to the respondents, specialty training provided the greatest amount of knowledge and skills used in their clinical practices, with a median contribution of 20%. Practice phase 2 was of great importance, with a median of 15% for those 75 responding physicians who had to attend it in 1989 or later. The education provided in medical school accounted for 15%. Preclinical education and formal CME each were given the lowest value, 5%, which is less than one-third of that given for practice-based learning.

The distributions of the percentages assigned to the individual phases show great variability. While the answers for preclinical education (range 0–30%), CME (range 0–30%), and practical year (range

0–40%) fall in a narrow range between 0 and 40%, only one or two answers have values at the upper border of the range. The answers for the other four phases have much larger ranges of gain, between 60% and 90%, as stated previously.

Sixty-nine of the 114 respondents (61%) said that one or more of the seven educational phases had made no contribution to their knowledge or skills. For preclinical education, 19 physicians (17% of the 114 who responded) said there had been no contribution; for clinical education, 10 (9%); for the practical year, 3 (3%); for practice phase 2, 17 (22% of the 75 having to attend it); for specialty training 16 (14%); for formal CME, 26 (23%); and for practice-based learning, 3 (3%). Thirty-six of the respondents saw no contribution from more than one phase up to a maximum of no contribution from four phases. Practice-based learning was only included once as noncontributory. On the other hand, many respondents perceived a contribution of 50% or more from one training phase: 2 indicated clinical education in medical school; 1, the practical year in a teaching hospital; 2, practice phase 2, and 23, specialty training. Six physicians stated that they had learned between 50% and 90% from independent learning after the conclusion of their postgraduate training. We found a significant difference in the participation in informal study groups depending on the year of licensure. Of the 38 respondents whose licenses were issued in 1985 or earlier, 21 (55%), including all 18 with board certification, answered that they were participating more or less regularly in study groups, compared with 23 (30%) of the 76 who had been licensed after 1986 ($p < .05$).

DISCUSSION

Our study's self-evaluation approach should show whether new insight can be gained into the relative contributions of the seven phases of physicians' total medical education as seen from the practice perspective. According to the answers from the 114 practicing physicians, 15% of the competencies used in the practice of medicine five years after the completion of postgraduate training were estimated to have been acquired in medical school, compared with 45% obtained from formal postgraduate education. The low rating for university education may have reflected the necessity to fill gaps in knowledge not learned successfully in medical school or physicians' updating themselves about recent scientific knowledge and clinical experience. This distribution may be supported by the efficacy of independent practice-based learning, which was rated as providing a learning contribution of 18%. The conditions for learning basic sciences in a structure that permits the knowledge to be used immediately for solving clinical problems are better during postgraduate training.

In the past, studies have dealt with special issues such as the relationship between achievement in medical school and measures of postgraduate performance.[45] Kassebaum pointed out that integrated analyses are few, longitudinal studies are rare, and use of the information gained in these studies to revise the undergraduate curriculum is limited.[88] The wide variations in the kinds of physicians' practices are often beyond the experience of those who define the curriculum. But undergraduate education must also confer a common knowledge base upon all doctors. The authors of a Finnish study[99] assessed the quality of different educational issues during undergraduate education and found a need for more emphasis on postgraduate vocational training and continuing education, including problem-oriented courses.

The findings of the present study may have been influenced by the quality of teaching typical of German physicians' medical education, but the conclusions from other investigations of the knowledge structure at the end of undergraduate education and its limited usefulness for problem solving are based on research carried out in the United Kingdom, Canada, and the United States. Awareness of the need to continue physicians' education beyond the undergraduate phase is common to all these countries. Our findings support the recommendation of Taylor that faculties should no longer behave as if their graduates had to learn in medical school all they will need for the practice of medicine.[175]

The striking diversity in the percentages of the contributions allotted to the seven phases of their education by the 114 physicians in this study shows that learning is a highly variable process and also illustrates the individuality of the physicians and their learning styles and learning environments, even assuming that subjective, perhaps even emotional, factors influenced these physicians' responses. According to their answers, the smallest contributions, often given as zero, had been provided by preclinical education and formal CME. In addition, 16 participants stated that they had learned nothing during specialty training. This is not plausible, but it may reflect the lack of teaching that often prevails in specialty training in Germany.

CONCLUSION

In spite of the limitations of this kind of survey, it seems worth the effort to improve on the method for further investigations; for example, by concentrating on physicians who have undergone uniform phases of education and who have practiced for at least five years since their board certification. The participants should be well informed about the issues and the definition of the education categories and should be highly motivated to participate in this form of study and to give accurate ratings.[92]

CHAPTER TWELVE

Examination of Nonresponse Bias in a Major Residency Follow-up Study

Steven J. Verhulst, Ph.D., and
Linda H. Distlehorst, Ph.D.

Survey instruments, used for both student and program evaluation in medical education, are also being used increasingly to evaluate residents' performances as a part of longitudinal institutional assessment. Several medical schools operate extensive residency follow-up programs that collect both objective and subjective evaluations of residents' performances during at least the first year of residency.[106,189] However, survey procedures or other factors can result in some instruments' not being returned, leading to the possible problem that the returned evaluations could be different from those evaluations not returned.[129] This problem is often referred to as nonresponse bias.

With most survey studies, the primary source of nonresponse bias is in the form of poor return rates and missing data.[4] To counter these omissions, response rates of 75% or higher have been recommended as necessary to avoid the effects of nonresponse bias.[58]

Another important source of nonresponse bias in residency evaluation is that of obtaining permission from medical students, who must provide written permission for their residency supervisors to be solicited for evaluation of their performances. Whether or not permission to collect supervisors' evaluation forms has been granted may have a severe effect on the school's interpretation and use of the evaluations for curriculum planning.

The purpose of this study was to examine the potential effects of these two types of nonresponse bias on supervisors' evaluations of residents' performances. In the context of this study, the first type of nonresponse bias is possible when residency supervisors do not return the residents' evaluation forms. As previously stated, the second type of bias is possible when medical students do not give the medical school permission to do follow-up evaluations of their performances in residencies. In order to evaluate the potential effects of these different types of nonresponse bias, residents who gave permission for follow-up and residents who did not give permission were compared on a number of standard measures collected during medical school. Similarly, supervisors who returned evaluation forms and supervisors who did not return forms were compared using the same measures.

METHOD

The Residency Follow-up Project has been in existence since 1975, when the members of Southern Illinois University School of Medicine's (SIU's) first graduating class entered their first year of residency. Each year in the late spring of the graduates' first residency year, the supervisors of all those graduates who have granted permission for follow-up receive the follow-up instrument at their institutions. The instrument is a 13-item survey questionnaire, where each item is to be rated on a ten-point scale (1=unsatisfactory; 10=outstanding). A more detailed account of the instrument is available elsewhere.[136] Follow-up letters and materials are provided after a three-week period in order to increase response rate.

For the purposes of this study, analyses were performed using residency follow-up evaluations for the combined classes of 1981 through 1988 to identify the response groups. To assess the impact of nonresponse bias, other measures were compared: grade-point averages (GPAs), scores on the Medical College Admission Test (MCAT), scores on the National Board of Medical Examiners (NBME) Part I and Part II examinations, results from the postclerkship examinations, race, and gender.

Of the 508 residents from the 8 SIU classes studied, 440 (87%) had given permission for obtaining their residency supervisors' evaluations. Of these 440 residents, there were 415 whose supervisor evaluation forms were returned (group 1), and 25 whose forms were not returned (group 2); overall, 82% of the residents' forms were returned (that is, the supervisor response rate was 82%). The 68 residents who did not give permission constitute group 3. The design employed was a one-factor analysis of variance (ANOVA), which consisted of the three levels identified by group above. To specifically test for the effect of permission, a linear contrast was applied to compare those who gave permission with those who did not give permission (group 1 and group 2 against group 3). Similarly, to test for the effect of supervisors' actions, a contrast was designed to compare the returns-with-permission group with the no-returns-with-permission group (group 1 against group 2). In addition to tests of significance, measures of effect size were also calculated. These effect sizes were calculated as the difference between the pooled means of group 1 and group 2 minus the mean of group 3 divided by the pooled standard deviation of group 1 and group 2. As suggested by Cohen[27], acceptable comparative values for small, medium, and large effect sizes could be .20, .50, and .80, respectively, for this study. Statistical significance was set at the .05 probability level, although values less than .1 are presented in Table 12.1.

RESULTS

The contrast comparing the permission groups (groups 1 and 2) with the no-permission group (group 3) indicates that the mean values of almost all the measures for the residents in the permission groups were significantly larger than those for the residents in the no-permission group. Specifically, the mean MCAT scores for all subtests were significantly higher for those residents providing permission than for those not doing so ($p < .05$). The results of the NBME Part I examination indicate that those residents who provided permission had significantly larger means on the NBME Part I total score as well as all the subscale scores except anatomy and microbiology. The NBME Part II scores showed no significant difference except for pediatrics, which was higher. In addition, postclerkship examination performances were not significantly different ($p = .055$) between permission groups (groups 1 and 2) (Table 12.1).

In general, the results for the supervisors who were given permission and who returned evaluation forms showed that 19 of 25 ($p < .007$) comparisons had larger means for returns than no returns (group 1 versus group 2) although only GPAs showed a statistically significant difference ($p < .02$). In addition, statistical analyses indicated that both the gender and the racial-ethnic group of the residents were significantly associated with permission. (For gender, $x^2 = 8.05$; $p < .018$; $df = 2$. For racial-ethnic group, $x^2 = 41.6$; $p < .001$; $df = 2$.) Specifically, the women and underrepresented-minority residents (American Indian, black, Mexican, and Puerto Rican) were less likely to

Table 12.1 Results of Analyses of Comparison Measures for Residents' Supervisors' Evaluations

Measure	Group 1 (n = 415) Permission with Return	Group 2 (n = 25) Permission with No Return	Group 3 (n = 68) No Permission with No Return	Group 1 + 2 with 3	
				Contrast p-values*	Effect Size
Grade-point average	(n = 393)	(n = 21)	(n = 68)		
Science	3.40	3.17	3.16	.107	.52
All other	3.56	3.42	3.44	ns	.28
Cumulative	3.46	3.23	3.28	.203	.45
MCAT†	(n = 392)	(n = 19)	(n = 68)		
Biology	9.45	9.84	8.65	.0005	.53
Chemistry	9.19	9.42	8.15	.0001	.68
Physics	9.15	9.47	8.01	.0001	.65
Science Problems	9.40	9.74	8.22	.0001	.82
Reading	8.90	8.68	8.21	.0432	.42
Quantitative	8.86	8.05	7.65	.0123	.65
NBME I‡	(n = 303)	(n = 19)	(n = 53)		
Anatomy	465	450	425	.0626	.41
Physiology	467	456	411	.0082	.56
Biochemistry	444	443	407	.0357	.38
Pathology	488	486	423	.0010	.65
Microbiology	428	424	395	.0938	.33
Pharmacology	510	518	445	.0001	.68
Behavioral Science	486	489	418	.0003	.66
Total Part I	463	458	399	.0009	.65

Measure	Group 1 ($n = 415$) Permission with Return	Group 2 ($n = 25$) Permission with No Return	Group 3 ($n = 68$) No Permission with No Return	Group 1 + 2 with 3	
				Contrast *p*-values*	Effect Size
NBME II[§]	($n = 295$)	($n = 18$)	($n = 36$)		
Medicine	483	474	449	ns	.38
Surgery	522	515	506	ns	.17
Ob/Gyn	516	496	502	ns	.16
Public Health	486	465	449	ns	.42
Pediatrics	504	497	462	.0379	.46
Psychiatry	494	474	460	ns	.35
Total Part II	500	482	463	ns	.43
Postclerkship	($n = 144$)	($n = 7$)	($n = 54$)		
Examination	69.6	67.6	66.7	.0550	.69

*Only p values <0.1 are presented, everything else is nonsignificant (ns).
†Medical College Admission Test score.
‡National Board of Medical Examiners Part I examination score.
§National Board of Medical Examiners Part II examination score.

provide permission to do follow-up evaluations of their performances as residents.

DISCUSSION

The supervisor response rate (82%) of SIU's Residency Follow-up Project clearly conforms to commonly recommended rates needed to avoid the effects of nonresponse bias. More important, however, this study clearly suggests that the effect of whether or not a medical student grants permission for the school to obtain residency follow-up information is critical to the interpretation, usefulness, and believability of the returned evaluations. However, the effects of whether or not a supervisor returns an evaluation form seems to have virtually no impact on information obtained through residency follow-up, provided the response rate is fairly high (as in this study).

Underrepresented-minority residents were less likely to have provided permission to obtain supervisor ratings when compared with majority (Hispanic, Asian, white) residents, and women residents were less likely to have provided permission to obtain supervisor rating forms. This might indicate that residency tracking, at least at SIU, needs to devote time and resources toward developing better relations and support networks for the underrepresented-minority and women students to foster productive, ongoing relationships.

The results clearly indicate that those residents providing permission had consistently higher GPAs and MCAT and NBME Part I scores, showing that the effect of granting permission was clearly discriminating for these measures. The influence of this discrimination is reflected in the effect sizes presented in Table 12.1. The effect sizes for significant variables ranged from .33 to .82. The average effect size for MCAT was .63 and that for NBME Part I was .52, demonstrating approximately six tenths of a standard deviation difference between means, a significant and sizable difference that suggests that who gives permission does contribute to a nonresponse bias, which should be considered when interpreting the results of the residency follow-up study. On the other hand, the effects on NBME Part II and the postclerkship examination score were not discriminating.

An interesting observation is that the nonresponse bias seemed to vanish for the NBME Part II scores, with an average effect size of approximately .32. This finding may have to do with the homogeneity of training in the clinical years, and with the clinical emphasis or the high pass rate on NBME Part II. The results for the postclerkship examination are also intriguing. Even though the mean for the postclerkship examination for those who provided permission was larger than the mean for the no-permission group, and the effect size (.69) was large, the finding was not statistically significant, although the difference was in the hypothesized direction. Intuitively, one would speculate that residents who do the poorest on the postclerkship examination would be least likely to provide permission to collect their supervisors' ratings.

Regarding the comparison of supervisors who returned and did not return the evaluations, the results indicate that for those residents who provided permission, only science GPA and cumulative GPA showed differences between the returns and no-returns. Returns were associated with GPAs about a quarter of a point higher than those associated with no-returns. No other significant effect was found, although many means were slightly larger for the return group, strongly supporting the view that there is very little, if any, bias attributable to supervisors' evaluations not being returned. Therefore, even though a lot of time may be devoted to collecting every supervisor evaluation, the direct reward for this investment is probably quite limited in terms of attributable bias.

Perhaps greater effort should be expended by the medical school to develop and maintain good "public relations" with its students so that its graduates feel a camaraderie toward their school and willingly participate in its institutional studies. This would help ensure that bias-free data are collected. The importance of obtaining permission to collect residency follow-up evaluations seems paramount if these evaluations are to be used to enhance or change the medical curriculum.

A larger leap, though a practical extension of these findings, would be to develop a procedure that would provide the medical school an estimate of the supervisors' ratings for the nonrespondents, based on the means of the respondents' ratings and the effect size derived from historical data. In addition, based on our experience, we would recommend that the medical students' permissions be collected early in the first year of medical school and that a form be used in which the student has to actively allow or not allow the collection of these data.

CHAPTER THIRTEEN

Measuring and Predicting the Performances of Practicing Physicians: An Overview of Two Decades of Research at the University of Utah

Calvin W. Taylor, Ph.D., and
Dominic Albo, Jr., M.D.

Essential to refinement of the selection and schooling of medical students is a clearer appreciation of the kind of physicians medical schools are trying to produce; that is, a more definite concept, for each medical specialty, of what performance criteria are implicit in the term "an excellent physician."

These elements of physicians' performances and medical school predictors of their performances were investigated on a small scale in the 1950s, when the first author carried out a study, sponsored by the Association of American Medical Colleges, of the predictive value of medical students' interviews. The first large-scale, comprehensive research into this matter was begun in the early 1960s—and resumed later in the 1970s—by a team of researchers (of which the authors were members) at the University of Utah School of Medicine. We were assembled and first directed by the late dean, Philip B. Price, former chairman of the Department of Surgery and also chairman of the medical school's admission committee. This article presents an overview of the major investigations in the 1960s and 1970s and the team's findings. More detailed descriptions of the studies and their results can be found elsewhere.[6,103,142,144–147,177,178]

THE INITIAL 1960s STUDY

Our initial study was undertaken with the premise that analysis of the performances of physicians in practice is an extremely complex matter, and that such performances are not susceptible to unidimensional measurement.[145] With this premise in mind, four types of physicians were studied: (1) 102 full-time faculty, of whom 73 were primarily clinicians and 29 were chiefly basic science teachers and investigators; (2) 190 board-certified urban specialists in practice, most of whom were also part-time members of the medical school's faculty; (3) 110 urban general practitioners; and (4) 105 rural and small-town general practitioners. This pool of 507 physicians was created to be a diverse and representative one that included physicians who had many types of practices and who were from a variety of social, economic, and professional environments; were from all adult age groups; and were graduates of many different medical schools with a variety of hospital training backgrounds.

Method

To develop a research instrument for measuring the physicians' performances, the team collected a large amount of information about each of these physicians from a variety of standard written records and from polls of medical students, department chairmen, and others associated with the physicians. Also, they asked the physicians themselves to fill out questionnaires and to participate in unhurried structured personal interviews conducted by experienced interviewers, wherein open-ended and provocative questions were posed and ample opportunity was provided for frank discussion and the expression of candid views. In addition, with each physician's permission, we obtained the confidential transcripts of his or her performances in college and medical school. All information collected about each physician was placed in a folder that was identified by a code number only.

Using this vast amount of raw data, the team identified over 200 different measures of practicing physicians' performances; some were common to the physicians in all four groups; others applied only to those in particular groups. The team subjectively selected for each group 80 measures that seemed particularly pertinent to that group. This number was dictated by the capacity of the mainframe computer being used at that time.

The team then used appropriate statistical methods to transform the large amount of complex and sometimes seemingly unrelated information they had collected into a manageable form. First, a standard scaling technique was used to convert the performance measures to "standardized scores," which would be used to evaluate each physician's performance. Next, the degrees of relationship between the individual performance measures were determined by computing coefficients of correlation, after which the patterns of intercorrelations among the 80 variables in each group were analyzed to isolate clusters of variables; each cluster was relatively independent of the others. Using factor analysis, the large number of variables was then reduced to a limited number of factors (i.e., categories) that could be interpreted in terms of their underlying characteristics.

These statistical manipulations enabled the team to present a representative profile of the performance of each physician studied. Each profile could be used to show how well each physician scored on each of the factors appropriate to the physician and his or her group.[144]

Findings

A prominent finding was that, as suspected, the analysis of physicians' practice performances is an extremely complex undertaking. For that reason, it would not suffice to categorize a physician as simply "good" or "poor" when assessing his or her overall accomplishments and contributions. Instead, it is necessary to determine the natures of the different aspects of the physician's performance on a complex multidimensional profile.

Another finding was the clear demonstration that the physician's performances during their formal education, as measured by grade-point averages (GPAs), constituted a factor that was almost completely independent of all the factors associated with their performances as physicians. This was true for the physicians in all four groups studied.

Specifically, the hundreds of intercorrelations were viewed across: (1) the measures of the physicians' academic performances (i.e., GPAs in their first two years of medical school), and (2) the 77 measures of their on-the-job performances; this process of comparison was repeated using the GPAs in their last two years of medical school. Ninety-seven percent of these intercorrelations were of a zero-order (.00) magnitude. Conversely, only 3% were large enough to indicate any significant relationship between the physicians' GPAs in medical school and their later performances in practice, and more of these intercorrelations were negative than positive. In fact, further computations indicated that the relation of the academic achievement measures and the performance measures is virtually the same as what would occur if the relation were a random one; the deviation from a random relation is mostly on the side of negative correlations.[144,147] For those who might argue that the lack of correlations shown between the physicians' academic performances at medical school and their practice performances were due to "restriction of range," the team included in their report of findings a technical explanation of why that influence was relatively unimportant (see Price and colleagues, pp. 98–118[145]).

The lack of relation between medical school performances and practice performances that the team found was "somewhat shocking" to the team, and their later report[144] discussed some of the issues about admission policies and conventional grades that were raised by this finding. Another important finding was that "a highly trained professional group—in this case, physicians—is amenable to analytical study, and that meaningful criterion data can be collected from them . . . that can be studied in a single integrated project. Although this research paradigm has been exploratory in nature . . . it provides a basis of orientation upon which future research can be built in a systematic manner."[144]

A LATER STUDY

In the early 1970s the team again studied physicians' performances and their relations to two criterion targets: their performances as medical students in their academic years (one and two) and their clinical years (three and four).[103]

Method

The first phase of this investigation was to discover what qualities define a "good physician," and how to turn these qualities into measures of the criterion targets. A list of 363 qualities of physicians was generated by 372 practicing physicians. These qualities were rated on the basis of their importance to superior physician performance by 85 other physicians, 84 medical students and residents, 162 college students, 98 nurses, 31 paramedical personnel, 855 randomly sampled members of the general public less than 65 years old, 35 persons 65 years old or older, and 267 persons from other groups (i.e., 89 blacks, 53 members of the 1960s counterculture, and 125 persons of low socioeconomic status).

The list of qualities was refined to create 87 positive qualities deemed necessary for superior performance and 29 characteristics seen as possibly detrimental to superior performance. More about these two lists is reported elsewhere.[146] The next challenge was to develop various rating forms by using the lists of positive and detrimental qualities.

As part of this step, conceptually homogeneous categories that allowed the qualities to be rated with composite scores were generated (using factor analysis) from the 363 items describing physicians' qualities. A panel of psychologists and physicians independently sorted these items into the following 11 categories of a physician's performance: (1) diagnostic-therapeutic knowledge, skills, and performance; (2) keeping abreast; (3) effectiveness in communicating with and instructing others; (4) quality of business practices; (5) human relations qualities in working with other health professionals; (6) general human relations qualities in dealing with patients; (7) general intellectual characteristics; (8) physical endurance; (9) ethics and character; (10) altruistic dedication to medicine; and (11) negative characteristics.

In addition to the items in these 11 categories, 10 items were selected from those used in the first 1960s study, including history-taking, physical examination, diagnosis, therapy, use of hospital, keeping abreast, and similar items. These ten items across five types of judges were treated as 50 categories. (The judges were house officers nurses, patients, physician observers, and—using self-evaluation—the physician himself or herself.) In this way, 61 categories (i.e., 50 + 11) that could be rated by composite scores were generated.

Then 167 Utah physicians were rated on these 62 categories. The 5 different types of judges were used to evaluate physician-quality items within their areas of expertise. (On 98 of the qualities, the physicians being studied evaluated themselves.) The physician plus a maximum of five judges of each of the other four types of judges provided ratings for each physician. The resulting form filled out for each physician contained 363 items of information.

Results

The results of this study showed the usefulness of a multiobserver, multimeasure approach to the assessment of physicians' performances. Correlations between the 167 physicians' medical school grades during all four years and the 61 composite performance scores ranged from −.25 to .25, with a median correlation of .02. Of the 61 validity correlations generated, only 3 reached significance at the .05 level. In addition, for the two clinical years of the physicians' grades and performances, the median correlation was −.03. Correlations were essentially .00 regardless of the source of the rating data (e.g., patients) and regardless of the particular composite of job performance being predicted.

The next analysis classified the Utah physicians by specialty: surgery, pediatrics, internal medicine, urban general practice, and rural general practice. The numbers of physicians in the individual specialties ranged from 22 to 34. For each specialty, the median correlations between premedical and medical school grades as predictors of the 61 performance measures for the specialty were obtained. Again, any relationships between such grades and the physicians' performances were nonsignificant across all five medical specialty groups.

The final analysis classified all the physicians by years of experience, grouped within intervals of 7 years (e.g., there were 28 physicians who had practiced at least 1 and as many as 7 years, 28 who had practiced at least 8 and as many as 14 years, etc.). For each group (without regard to specialty), two sets of validity correlations were computed for each measure of academic achievement as predictors of on-the-job performance. Again, the physicians' medical school grades were not significantly related to their performance scores, no matter what the levels of their experience.

CONCLUSION

The studies described in this article indicate that the total complex array of talents and skills that are needed for a physician to perform effectively are poorly measured by academic achievement scores, which tap only a very narrow band of the extremely complex total spectrum of skills, abilities, and performances of practicing physicians. It is clear that in comparison with the great complexity of the performances of practicing physicians, the selection and educational processes in medical schools are remarkably simple and to a large degree not directed to or relevant to fostering many of the multiplicity of skills the practicing physician needs.

THE FUTURE

As we see it, the most challenging research work ahead is to produce more wide-range, complex selection and performance measures that have useful predictive value. The best type of measuring device that we have found is the well-constructed, refined, and validated biographical inventory.[177,178]

In terms of improving the training of physicians, we think that the quickest and easiest approach would be to work with physicians-in-training (residents), because most residency activities can be designed to parallel at an earlier stage the performances of physicians in practice.[5] We have pursued fruitful investigations on methods of teaching communication and fostering creativity, decision making, and other skills that could be useful in such training and that are already being taught to other kinds of students through programs funded by the Department of Education.[179]

The approaches just mentioned are the ways that medicine can use to greatly enlarge the human capabilities of students going through the full medical program to become physicians. In this way, schools will be fostering the complex attributes that will ultimately be required of their students as practicing physicians.[176]

ACKNOWLEDGMENTS

The research reported in this paper could not have come about without the creative vision and hard work of the late dean Philip B. Price. Others physicians who have been important in the various investigations that have taken place over the years are J. Gary Maxwell, Frank G. Moody, Hugh H. Hogle, William Gay, and Patrick Bray. Others who were important in the work when they were completing their doctoral degrees are James M. Richards, Jr., David E. Nelson, Brent Page, Stanley A. Mulaik, and Alan Lau. The authors especially thank those organizations that funded the project at various times, especially Robert Beezer, who provided the first major funding that launched this research effort.

CHAPTER FOURTEEN

Is the Glass Half Full or Half Empty? A Reexamination of the Associations Between Assessment Measures During Medical School and Clinical Competence After Graduation

Mohammadreza Hojat, Ph.D.,
Joseph S. Gonnella, M.D., J. Jon Veloski, M.S.,
and James B. Erdmann, Ph.D.

Determining the associations between the knowledge and skills acquired in professional education and performance in practice has always been a challenge to researchers. Investigating the issue is particularly important in medicine because of the economic and social implications. Given the magnitudes of the investments by both students and the government in medical education, medical school curricula should be relevant to elements of the practice domain for economic reasons. At the same time, medical schools should be committed to assuring that the students and residents who ultimately serve the public are armed with knowledge and skills they need to render optimum service. To achieve these goals there is a need to establish the associations between assessments of knowledge, skills, and competence in medical school and after graduation.

Empirical investigations of these associations have produced inconsistent and ambiguous findings. Although it is customary to highlight previous empirical findings, we instead refer readers to the introductory article of this monograph to avoid redundancy (see "A Case of Mistaken Identity"). In that article, we present a comprehensive review of the literature on the topic and discuss the "signals" that contribute to perception of the strengths of the relationships and the "noises" that obscure them. In particular, the conceptual and methodologic issues discussed in that section have important relevance to the present study in both the statements of hypotheses and the method used to analyze the data.

The present study was designed to reexamine the connections between measures of academic performance during medical school and those obtained one year after graduation from medical school by applying appropriate methods of statistical analysis and by employing homogeneously derived measures of performance. We tested the following research hypotheses:

1. Objective measures of medical knowledge attained during medical school and one year after graduation are highly correlated.
2. Students' low or high academic standings in medical school are directly and significantly associated with their subsequent clinical competence ratings as residents.
3. The association between academic standings in medical school and status on clinical competence ratings as residents is stronger for measurements that are conceptually more similar than dissimilar.

In addition, based on previous findings,[45] we investigated the strengths of associations in different postgraduate training areas and at different levels of performance.

METHODS AND PROCEDURES

The following methods and procedures were used.

Methods

Data Sources

Data on performances during medical school, in residency, and in practice for a cohort of graduates were retrieved from the database of the Jefferson longitudinal study of medical students and graduates.

Survey Sample

The total sample consisted of 2,368 graduates of Jefferson Medical College between 1980 and 1990. Scores on Part III of the National Board of Medical Examiners (NBME) examinations were available for the 1,779 graduates (75% of the total sample) who had given written permission for collecting them. While a similar proportion of graduates (75%) had given permission to collect data from their postgraduate training program directors, usable postgraduate rating forms were received for only 1,724 graduates (73% of the total sample).

Measures of Academic Performance During Medical School

Grades earned in the following major courses in the first three years of medical school were: *freshman year*—anatomy, biochemistry, histology, mechanisms of disease, and physiology (five variables); *sophomore year*—introduction to clinical medicine, microbiology, pathology, and pharmacology (four variables); *junior year*—examination grades in the six required core clerkships (family medicine, internal medicine, obstetrics–gynecology, pediatrics, psychiatry, and surgery) and the global ratings of clinical competence in each of these six clerkships.

Altogether, 21 measures of academic performance in medical school were chosen for this study (objective examinations at Jefferson have acceptable internal consistency, indicated by reliability coefficients around .75). Because of the elective nature of the senior-year clerkships and the variation in the assessments, no evaluation measure for this year was included in the study. Also, total scores on Part I (knowledge of sciences basic to medicine) and Part II (knowledge of clinical sciences) of the NBME examinations were chosen as additional measures of academic attainment in medical school.

Measures of Postgraduate Clinical Competence

The assessment of postgraduate clinical competence was obtained from the director of each graduate's training program or the physician most familiar with the resident's performance. The evaluator was asked to respond to 33 statements by giving ratings on a four-point Likert-type scale. These assessments were performed at the end of the first postgraduate training year to give the evaluator ample time to observe the resident. For a more stable standard, the instructions emphasized that the evaluator should compare the resident with *all* the graduates the evaluator had supervised, not just those in the recent group. The order of appearance of the rating statements in the form was random, and the raters were asked to consider each item independently. Data are available to support the measurement characteristics and psychometric properties of the Jefferson postgraduate rating form.[66,68,72,186,187] In addition to the ratings of clinical competence, scores on the objective examination of the NBME (Part III) were used as performance measures in residency. This examination measures clinical competence and patient management skills and is usually taken at the end of the first year of the residency training.

Procedures

The following procedures were employed to measure components of performance in medical school and after graduation.

Components of Performance Measures in Medical School

Data on academic performances in medical school obtained from course grades and clerkship ratings in medical school were subjected to factor analysis for more manageable statistical analysis. The factor-analytic study was performed on assessments conducted by Jefferson faculty. External examination scores (Parts I and II of the National Board) were not included in the factor-analytic study. The principal-components factor analysis was used, and orthogonal varimax rotation procedures was employed to simplify the obtained factor structure.

The factor analysis of the 21 academic performance measures resulted in 3 initial factors with eigenvalues greater than unity.[85] An examination of the initial factor pattern indicated that the 3 extracted factors accounted for 52% of the total covariance (factor I accounted for 35%, factor II for 10%, and factor III for 7%). Factor I, or the grand factor, represented all six objective clerkship examination grades in the junior year, grades in all four courses in the sophomore year, and the grade in the mechanisms of disease course in the freshman year. All these 11 variables had factor loadings greater than .50 on factor I (the highest loading was equal to .74 for the internal medicine clerkship examination). Factor I was entitled "sciences related to clinical medicine." All 5 freshman course grades had factor loadings of .80 or above on factor II (with factor loadings ranging from .79 to .82), entitled "sciences basic to medicine." The clinical competence ratings in the six junior clerkships loaded on the factor III with loading magnitudes between .67 (for family medicine clerkships) and .50 (for obstetrics–gynecology). Other variables had either zero or negligible loadings on this factor, which was called "clinical competence rating."

Based on the results of the factor analysis, composite scores of the variables that contributed to each of the three factors (sciences related to clinical medicine, sciences basic to medicine, and clinical competence ratings in medical school) were calculated and defined as the three components of academic performance in medical school for statistical analysis. The composite scores were calculated based on the unweighted sum of the variables with loadings above .50 on each factor.

Components of Postgraduate Competence Ratings

The residency directors' ratings on the 33 statements in the postgraduate rating form had been subjected to factor analysis previously and the results published.[68,72] Analysis of the 33 ratings yielded three factors: "data-gathering and processing skills" (the grand factor, accounting for 60% of the total covariance); "interpersonal and attitudinal" (5% of the total covariance); and "socioeconomic aspects of patient care" (4% of the total covariance). Detailed analyses and descriptions of rating statements, factor loadings, and other psychometric data are given elsewhere.[72] Construct and predictive validities of the factors have also been reported.[68] Factors similar to the first two factors have been reported in other factor-analytic studies of areas of postgraduate competence by Arnold and colleagues[8] and Dowaliby and Andrew.[33] To check the stability of the factors, the factor analysis of the postgraduate ratings was replicated using the sample of the present study. The results were found to be similar to the previous findings, and the factor loadings seemed especially like duplicate findings of those in the previous study. Therefore based on factor-analytic results, composite scores of ratings of statements contributing to each of the three factors were calculated, and, accordingly, three postgraduate competence components of "data-gathering and processing skills," "interpersonal and attitudinal," and "socioeconomic aspects of patient care" were defined as the areas of postgraduate competence.

Because the distributions of the ratings of postgraduate competence and their composite measures are seriously skewed,[186,204] and the assumption of homoscedasticity does not hold with the rating data, we used distribution-free statistical methods when analyzing data on postgraduate competence ratings. Thus the sample was divided into three groups based on score distributions of the composite measures of components of academic performance in medical school and into another three groups based on score distributions of postgraduate competence areas (top quarter, middle half, and bottom quarter). The purpose was to investigate whether the students in the top and bottom quarters on the measures of performance in medical school would be located in the top and bottom quarters, respectively, of the distributions of the ratings of postgraduate competence areas. A particular research interest was to examine the proportions of the top quarter of medical students who were also rated among the top quarter of residents on postgraduate competence areas (true-positive rate, or sensitivity), and the proportions of the bottom quarter of medical students who were also rated among the bottom quarter of residents on postgraduate competence areas (true-negative rate, or specificity). Nonparametric inferential technique (chi-square) was applied. Since normality and homoscedasticity assumptions are not violated in using the scores of the NBME examinations and composite measures of clinical and basic sciences examination grades (the first two factors of academic performance in medical school), parametric statistical methods (e.g., Pearson product-moment correlation) were applied.

RESULTS AND DISCUSSION

We first analyzed the data to test the three hypotheses; then we conducted additional analyses in terms of the graduates' medical specialties and board certification.

Analysis

The following correlational analyses were performed to test the first research hypothesis that the objective measures of medical knowledge are correlated. The total scores on NBME Part II (an objective measure of knowledge of clinical sciences during medical school) were correlated with the total scores on NBME Part III (which purports to measure clinical decision making and patient management in residency). The correlation between Part II scores and Part III scores was .72 (p <.01). Also, the correlation between objective clinical examination grades in medical school and Part III scores was .59 (p <.01). These findings confirm the first hypothesis.

Additional correlational analyses were performed to examine the relationships between measures of achievement in basic sciences in medical school and Part III scores, with an expectation that these correlations should be lower than those reported above because of the time intervals between the testings and the content dissimilarities. The correlations between NBME Part I total scores and examination grades in basic sciences in medical school on the one hand and Part III scores on the other hand were .60 and .45, respectively. Both of these correlations were significantly lower than the corresponding correlations when objective clinical sciences performance measures were correlated with Part III (.72 for Parts II and III versus .60 for Parts I and III; and .59 for clinical examination grades and Part III versus .45 for examination grades in basic science and Part III). The correlations between examination grades in medical school (in both basic and clinical sciences) and Part III scores were lower than corresponding correlations with the NBME Part I and Part II scores despite the fact that all of these examinations use the same multiple-choice-question format (except the family medicine clinical examination, which has a short-essay format). Differences in psychometric characteristics of the local examinations at Jefferson and the standardized examinations developed by the NBME could account for the correlational differences.

The following analyses were performed to test the second research hypothesis concerning associations between students' low or high academic standings in medical school and high or low standings on ratings of clinical competence in residency.

Correlational analyses do not seem appropriate when skewed distributions of ratings are considered. It has been reported that the correlations cannot attain their maximal values when the distributions are skewed.[23,69] Therefore categorical analyses were performed on the top-quarter, middle-half, and bottom-quarter groups.

Percentage distributions of the groups in these three categories (based on composite measures of performances in medical school and ratings in the area of data-gathering and processing skills) are presented in Table 14.1.

The data show several patterns. First, the likelihood of being rated in the bottom quarter on data-gathering and processing skills in residency was much higher (almost twice as high) for the physicians who performed in the bottom quarter of the performance scale in medical school than for those in the top quarter. For example, 35% (141) of those in the bottom quarter of the scale for basic sciences examinations were also rated in the bottom quarter of postgraduate ratings of data-gathering and processing skills, while only 20% (82) of those in the bottom quarter of the scale for basic sciences examinations were rated in the top quarter of postgraduate ratings. These associations became stronger when relationships between global ratings of clinical competence in medical school and postgraduate competence ratings were examined (see Table 14.1).

Second, similar patterns can be observed in top-quarter performances. For example, 31% (142) of those in the top quarter of the scale for basic science examinations were also rated in the top quarter of postgraduate ratings of data-gathering and processing skills, while only 18% (85) of top scorers in medical school were rated in the bottom quarter of the rating scale in residency. Again, associations between performances in medical school and postgraduate ratings of clinical competence became stronger for clinical sciences examinations than basic sciences examinations in medical school, and they became strongest for global ratings of clinical competence in medical school and postgraduate ratings of competence.

Table 14.1 Percentage Distribution of 1,704 Graduates of Jefferson Medical College between 1980 and 1990 by Performance in Medical School and Postgraduate Ratings of Clinical Competence in Data-gathering and Processing Skills*

	Rating of Data-gathering and Processing Skills at the End of the First Year of Residency		
Medical School Performance	**Bottom Quarter (n = 416) (%)**	**Middle Half (n = 870) (%)**	**Top Quarter (n = 418) (%)**
Bottom quarter (n = 409)			
Basic sciences examinations	35	45	20
Clinical sciences examinations	37	45	18
Global ratings of competence	42	41	17
Middle half (n = 831)			
Basic sciences examinations	23	54	23
Clinical sciences examinations	23	54	23
Global ratings of competence	24	56	20
Top quarter (n = 464)			
Basic sciences examinations	18	51	31
Clinical sciences examinations	16	51	33
Global ratings of competence	14	49	37

*The authors examined the associations between measures of performance in medical school and ratings of clinical competence made by residency directors at the end of the first year of residency. For basic sciences examination grades, $\chi^2_{(4)} = 39.35$, $p < .01$; for clinical sciences examination grades, $\chi^2_{(4)} = 66.73$, $p < .01$; for global ratings of clinical competence in medical school, $\chi^2_{(4)} = 118.62$, $p < .01$.

These findings indicate that significant associations exist among all three performance measures in medical school and ratings of postgraduate clinical competence in data-gathering and processing skills.

Third, another pattern is related to a well-known statistical phenomenon, "regression toward the mean." As shown in Table 14.1, a great number of students who were in either top or bottom quarters of performance measures in medical school were rated in the middle group in their assessments in residency.

Patterns of the relationships between the three performance measures in medical school and two other measures of postgraduate clinical competence (interpersonal skills and attitudes, and socioeconomic aspects of patient care) were similar to those reported in Table 14.1, with two exceptions: basic sciences examination grades were not significantly associated with ratings on socioeconomic aspects of patient care, and the top-quarter students in medical school could not be significantly differentiated by ratings of postgraduate competence in interpersonal skills and attitudes. Almost equal proportions of students in the top quarter of the scale for basic sciences examinations in medical school were rated in the top and bottom quarters of this postgraduate clinical competence area (18% and 19%, respectively). As was noticed before, ratings of clinical competence in medical school yielded the strongest associations with all three areas of postgraduate clinical competence ratings.

The findings reported in Table 14.1 indicate that, in general, significant associations exist between measures of performance in medical school and ratings of postgraduate clinical competence in data-gathering and processing skills. In other words, the likelihood of being rated in the top quarter of competence in residency is higher for those who performed in the top quarter in the class in medical school than for their counterparts in the bottom quarter. Also, those whose performances in medical school placed them in the bottom quarter of the scale were likely to be rated accordingly in the bottom quarter of postgraduate competence ratings. The associations hold for all three performance measures in medical school: grades on basic science and clinical science examinations, and global ratings of clinical competence in junior core clerkships. The strengths of the associations varied for different areas of postgraduate competence, suggesting that the associations were stronger when performance measures in medical school and residency were conceptually similar (e.g., data-gathering and processing skills) than when they were dissimilar (e.g., socioeconomic aspects of patient care). These findings confirm the second and third research hypotheses.

The third hypothesis, concerning stronger associations between conceptually similar than dissimilar measures in medical school and residency, addresses this issue. The following analyses were performed to test the hypothesis further.

Specifically to investigate the associations between top- and bottom-quarter performers, we excluded the middle group and chose only those in the top and bottom quarters of performance scales and calculated proportions of "hits" and "misses." Those who were in the top quarter or bottom quarter of performance in medical school and were rated in the corresponding groups in the postgraduate clinical competence areas (top or bottom quarter) are defined as the "hits." On the contrary, those in the top or bottom quarters of performance in medical school who were rated in the opposite group in residency (top performers in medical school rated in the bottom quarter of the postgraduate clinical area and vice versa) were defined as "misses." The proportions of hits and misses for the three performance measures in medical school by ratings in different postgraduate clinical competence areas are presented in Figure 14.1A–C.

If the associations had been perfect (desirable but almost impossible in reality), all top graduates in medical school should have also been rated top in residency and vice versa (the proportions of hits and misses would be 100% and 0%, respectively); in such a case, there would be no bars in the upper-left and lower-right sections of the graphs. In a situation where associations were random, the bars would have equal heights in all four sections of each graph (assuming equal marginal frequencies). The proportions of hits or misses would be equally 50%.

Data reported in Figure 14.1A indicate that the proportion of hits is over 60% when the associations between the top and bottom quarters of the scale for basic sciences examinations in medical school and postgraduate clinical competence ratings on data-gathering and processing skills are considered. This proportion is higher (above 70%) when one examines the associations between the top and bottom quarters on global ratings of clinical competence in medical school and the corresponding groups based on the postgraduate clinical competence ratings. The proportions of misses are much smaller than the proportions of hits. The proportions of hits and misses for clinical sciences examinations lie somewhere between those for the basic sciences examinations and the global ratings in medical school. Thus, the data in Figure 14.1A provide evidence of associations between the three performance measures in medical school and clinical competence assessments in the area of data-gathering and processing skills in residency.

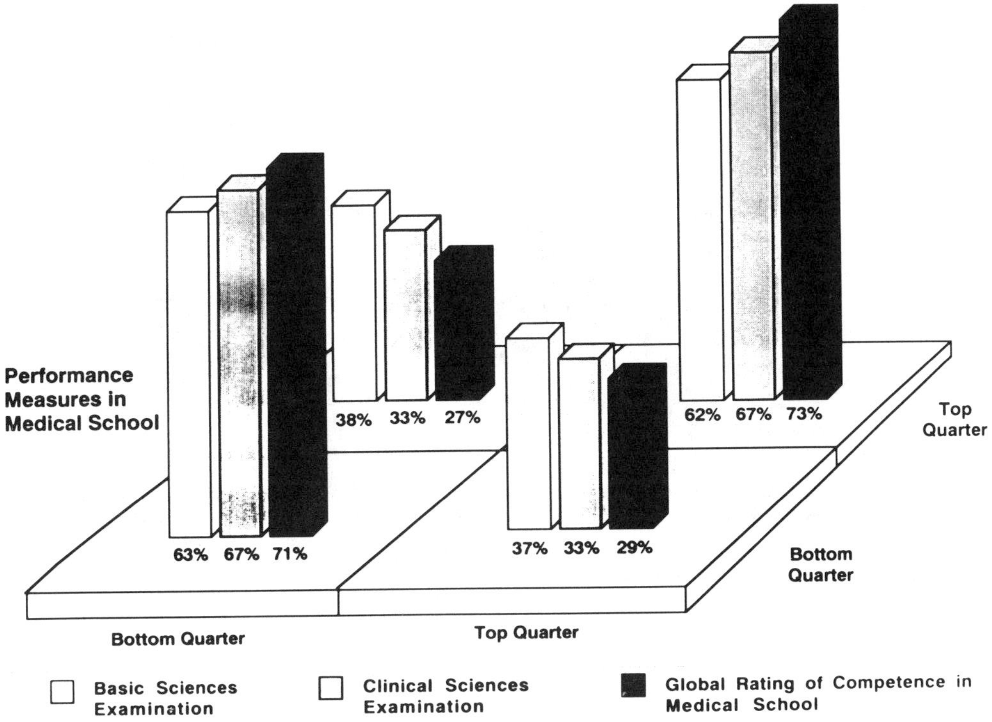

Figure 14.1A Performances in Medical School and Residency: Ratings of Data-Gathering and Processing Skills in Residency.

Figure 14.1B presents the associations between the three performance measures in medical school and the postgraduate competence ratings in the area of interpersonal skills and attitudes. As shown by the proportions of hits and misses, the association between the scale for basic science examinations and the postgraduate ratings becomes weaker than before, and the difference between the proportions of hits and misses, as reported previously, becomes nonsignificant for top-quarter scorers in medical school.

The associations between the scale for clinical sciences examinations and the global ratings of competence in medical school, on the one hand, and postgraduate competence ratings in the area of interpersonal skills and attitudes, on the other hand, become weaker (but still statistically significant) compared with corresponding proportions reported in Figure 14.1A. The proportion of hits for the global ratings of competence in medical school shows a slight improvement over the

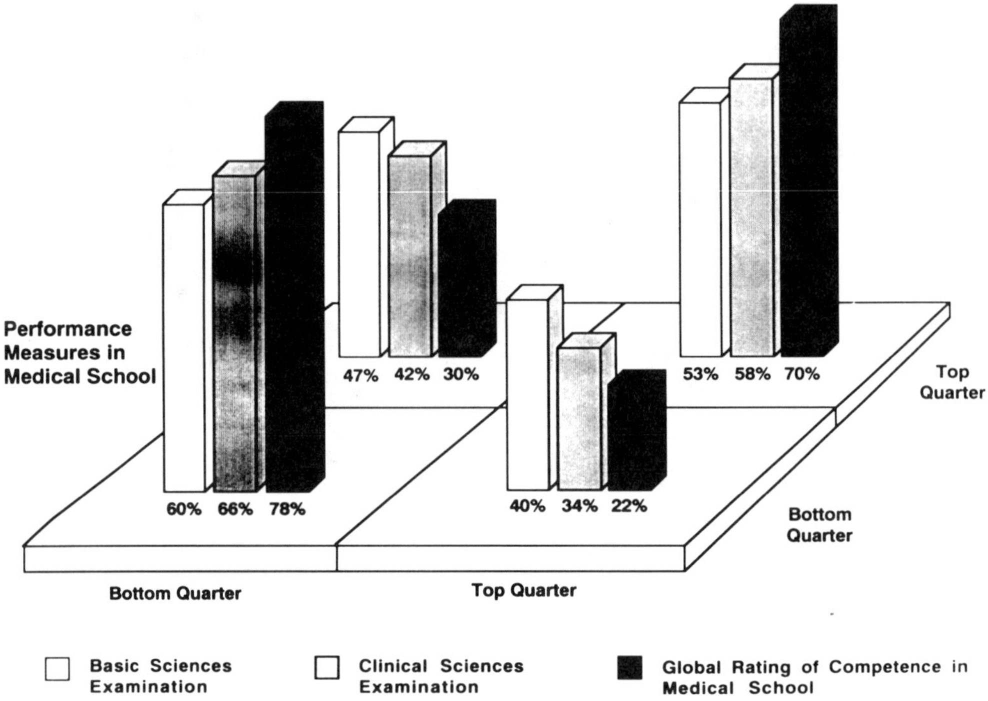

Figure 14.1B Performances in Medical School and Residency: Ratings of Interpersonal Skills and Attitudes in Residency.

corresponding proportion reported in Figure 14.1A for postgraduate competence ratings on data-gathering and processing skills.

Figure 14.1C presents data for the three performance measures in medical school by postgraduate competence ratings in socioeconomic aspects of patient care.

The proportions of hits and misses are similar to those in Figure 14.1B. The strongest association is for global ratings of clinical competence in medical school (70% proportion of hits), and the weakest association is for the basic science examinations (56% proportion of hits).

These findings confirm the third research hypothesis: conceptually similar assessments (e.g., global assessments of clinical competence in medical school and assessments of postgraduate clinical competence) were highly associated. One may attribute these associations to the similarity of the assessment formats, which could be confounded by halo effects. Our data indicate that this argument may be only partially true,

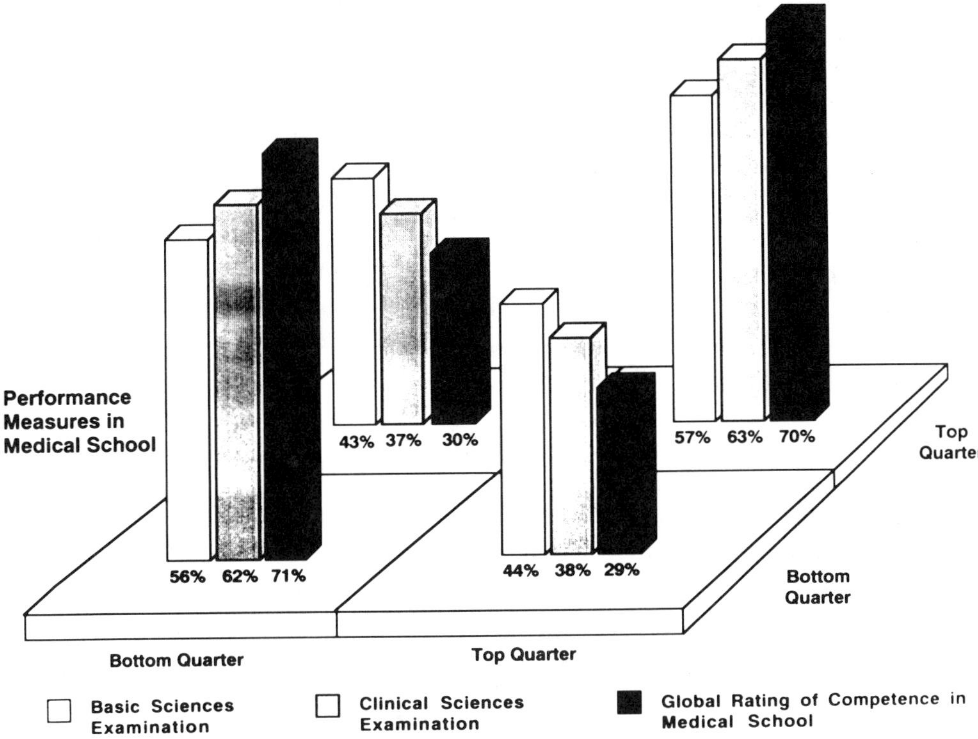

Figure 14.1C Performances in Medical School and Residency: Ratings of Socioeconomic Aspects of Patient Care in Residency.

since relatively strong associations were also observed when grades in objective examinations (in both the basic and the clinical sciences) were examined in relation to ratings of postgraduate competence in data-gathering and processing skills.

It can be reasonably assumed that postgraduate clinical competence in data-gathering and processing skills requires more acquired knowledge of basic and clinical sciences than, for example, postgraduate competence in socioeconomic aspects of patient care. The content of the rating statement used in the postgraduate ratings form attests to the fact that, indeed, statements such as "knowledge of basic science related to postgraduate program" are included among the items that assess data-gathering and processing skills. (For an examination of the content of the items in each area of postgraduate competence, see Table 14.1 in Hojat and colleagues' study.[72])

Based on these assumptions, one may expect a stronger association between conceptually related measures of grades on basic sciences and clinical sciences examinations in relation to postgraduate competence in data-gathering and processing skills, than in relation to the postgraduate competence in socioeconomic aspects of patient care. The data reported in Figure 14.1 confirm this expectation. The proportions of hits for the basic sciences and clinical sciences grades are higher in Figure 14.1A (for data-gathering and processing skills) than in Figure 14.1C (for socioeconomic aspects of patient care). These findings support the third research hypothesis.

Additional Analyses

In a previous study it was reported that the strengths of the associations between performances in medical school and ratings of postgraduate competence varied for graduates who had pursued different specialties.[45] To test the stability of that study's results, the strengths of the associations between performance measures in medical school and ratings of postgraduate clinical competence were examined for graduates in different postgraduate specialties. Five residency areas were chosen: internal medicine (n = 571), family practice (n = 331), surgery (n = 342), obstetrics–gynecology (n = 99), and pediatrics (n = 92). These specialty areas were chosen because of the relatively large numbers of graduates pursuing them. The associations between two performance measures in medical school (examination grades in basic sciences and global ratings of clinical competence in core clerkships) and postgraduate ratings in data-gatherings and processing skills were examined for each of these specialties. Stronger associations were found for those who had pursued internal medicine, obstetrics–gynecology, and surgery than for those in pediatrics and family medicine. Also, in internal medicine, family practice, and obstetrics–gynecology, the associations were stronger for those in the top quarters of their classes in global ratings of clinical competence than for their counterparts rated in the bottom quarters of their classes. On the contrary, for those who had pursued surgery and pediatrics, the associations were stronger for those who were rated in the bottom quarters of their classes in their core clerkships than for their counterparts rated in the top quarters of their classes.

The associations between basic sciences examination grades and postgraduate ratings on data-gathering and processing skills were statistically significant for those who had pursued internal medicine, obstetrics–gynecology, and surgery, but not for those who had chosen family practice and pediatrics. These findings confirm that the strengths of associations between performance measures in medical school and those in residency are a function of types of medical school performance measures (e.g., basic sciences examinations, global ratings of competence), levels of performance (top versus bottom quarter), and specialty. Consistent with previous findings,[45] our data indicate that the issue of associations between assessment measures in medical school and in practice is complex, and many factors should be taken into consideration in order to understand the relationships better.

Additional analyses were performed to investigate the board certification status of graduates who were in the top quarter, middle half, or bottom quarter of the medical school performance measures. These analyses were performed on 1,722 physicians who had graduated before 1988 (classes of 1980–1987) to allow sufficient time to complete residency training and become eligible for certification. Board certification was associated with the level of performance in medical school. For example, 65% (257) of those in the top quarter compared with 54% (459) in the middle half and to 51% (232) in the bottom quarter of the basic sciences examination scale were board certified ($\chi^2_{(2)} = 18.05$, $p < .01$).

CONCLUSION

The data presented in this report document that associations do exist between performance measures in medical school and those after graduation. Our findings indicate that performances during medical school and in residency are multidimensional concepts and that conceptually similar measures yield stronger associations than dissimilar ones. In addition, the strengths of associations varied for different performance measures and in different areas of specialization and at different levels of performance. The associations can be improved by refining the assessment instruments and considering the intervening variables described previously. Furthermore, in a recent study[70] as well as a previous one,[73] we observed that associations among performance measures in medical school increased drastically (more than 100% increment in R^2s) when selected measures of personality were added to the prediction models.

Our findings should give medical school faculty members confidence that their judgments are valid. While refinements should be sought, it is nonetheless appropriate for medical schools to focus especially on those students who perform marginally. These are the students who should be required to correct their deficiencies before they are graduated, since their future performances in general are a reflection of their past performances. Residency programs should pay attention to the performance dimensions that are more relevant to their objectives rather than to a single evaluation (e.g., class rank). Medical school faculty should concentrate on the students at the low end of the performance scale and propose remediation.

After all, what should be the response to the question in the title of this article: Is the glass half full or half empty? The truth is in the eye of the beholder—but the data presented here suggest that the glass is more than half full.

PART FOUR

Epilogue

Attempt the end, and never stand to doubt;
Nothing's so hard, but search will find out.

Robert Herrick
1591–1674

CHAPTER FIFTEEN

What Have We Learned, and Where Do We Go From Here?

Joseph S. Gonnella, M.D., Mohammadreza Hojat, Ph.D., James B. Erdmann, Ph.D., and J. Jon Veloski, M.S.

Medical colleges and the medical profession have always faced challenges. Each generation believes that its problems are unique, but many of today's issues are essentially the same as those faced by previous medical educators. They too had to select their medical students using limited information, design and implement curricula with finite resources, evaluate their educational programs, and monitor the performances of students. But the enormous sum of money that society is spending on medical education and health care is unique to our generation, and this has created a new crisis for the medical profession. To continue justifying an allocation of about 14% of our gross national product for these functions, the medical profession should be able to demonstrate that it is educating physicians who can translate their knowledge into performance, recognize their limitations, learn from their mistakes, keep up with advances in science and technology, and ultimately provide high-quality care at a reasonable cost for the patients they serve. Not all of these issues can be addressed in detail in a single monograph. We have attempted to explore one of them: Are knowledge and skills acquired in medical school translated into performance in practice?

Now that we have come so far on this journey, the logical questions are: *What have we learned ?* and *Where do we go from here?* Let us first reflect for a moment on what we have learned so far.

WHAT HAVE WE LEARNED?

All of the articles of this monograph except that of Taylor and Albo provide either conceptual reasons or empirical evidence that a continuity exists between assessments in medical school and those in practice. These reports present an optimistic view that our medical schools are educating physicians who perform in a manner consistent with the evaluations made in medical school. This is encouraging, and it indicates that there is validity to our educational activities and their assessments.

These results are observed despite the fact that some of the medical school achievement measures that are often considered one-dimensional are rather complex. For example, grade-point average (GPA) may seem straightforward and simple, but the GPA is not only made up of a variety of performance measures in several different disciplines but also the result of different standards, different methods of evaluation, and different content and skill specifications. It is not unreasonable to expect basic science performance to exhibit several dimensions, some determined by the different skills implicit in the assessments involved in various grades.

The reports include longitudinal data from five medical schools: the University of Missouri–Kansas City (Arnold and Willoughby), The Medical College of Georgia (Fincher and colleagues), Jefferson Medical College (Hojat and colleagues), Wright State University (Markert), and Southern Illinois University (Vu and colleagues). These analyses provide convincing evidence to refute criticism concerning external validity (generalizability), reliability (reproducibility), the effect size, and the lack of statistical power of the findings.

First, the issue of a lack of generalization of the findings can be rejected on the ground that the empirical data reported in this monograph were from five medical schools, public and private, in different geographic areas with varied educational programs and diverse populations of students and graduates. Evidence for external validity or generalizability of the findings is provided by the significant associations between performances before and after graduation from medical school that were consistently found for the graduates of all these medical schools.

Second, the similarities in the patterns of findings using longitudinal data from these institutions indicate that the findings are reproducible; hence, their reliability is supported. This monograph has provided an opportunity for several medical schools to use their longitudinal databases to address a specific issue of paramount importance, to test similar research hypotheses, and to use similar or comparable methods for

Table 15.1 Descriptive Data Selected from Empirical Studies Reported in This Monograph and Their Combined Analyses*

	Competence Ratings in Residency		
Medical School Performance	**Bottom-rated %**	**Top-rated %**	**No. of Trainees**
Top scorers			
Arnold and Willoughby	23	77	40
Fincher et al.	3	97	59
Hojat et al.	38	62	227
Markert	27	73	66
Vu et al.	12	88	117
Combined data	**25**	**75**	**509**
Bottom scorers			
Arnold and Willoughby	54	46	26
Fincher et al.	39	61	33
Hojat et al.	63	37	223
Markert	76	24	51
Vu et al.	38	62	16
Combined data	**61**	**39**	**349**

*Data were extracted from tables presented in the indicated studies reported in this monograph. Assessment measures in medical school and residency, and definition of top and bottom groups, are described in the text. Combined data are based on cumulative information from the selected studies.

data analyses, all leading to one conclusion. Although different assessment instruments and formats were used in the studies reported here, the methodologic similarities provide a unique opportunity to present a meta-analytic[126] review of the findings and power analyses of selected data for each institution and for all institutions combined.

In order to present a global picture of the findings from these medical schools, we extracted data from their results. Frequency data for the top and bottom groups of the articles by Arnold and Willoughby, Fincher and colleagues, Hojat and colleagues, Markert, and Vu and colleagues were extracted (Table 15.1). Percentage distributions and the numbers of observations on which the percentages were based for each study and for all studies combined are presented in Table 15.1.

A few points of caution should be made before describing the results. First, the predictors (independent variables), or performance measures during medical school, were not calculated based on a uniform assessment tool in all these studies. For example, in the Arnold and Willoughby study, the performance measure was represented by a factor called "knowledge" that included grade-point averages in medical school and the intramural quarterly profile examinations. In Hojat and colleagues' study, it was a composite score of basic sciences course grades in the first year of medical school, and in Vu and colleagues' study it was based on standardized patient-based postclerkship examinations given to the fourth-year students, and so forth. The dissimilarities in medical school assessment tools may limit the specific *conceptualization* of the variable, but for the purpose of *operationalization,* we may define it as a performance measure in medical school regardless of its format, specific contents, or chronologic administrations.

Second, the criterion measures (dependent variables), or ratings of clinical competence in residency, were calculated based on different rating forms with different number of items, which were completed by the directors of residency programs in the late months of the first postgraduate year. Again, this lack of uniformity of the assessment instruments limits, to some extent, the content specificity of the criterion measure, but for operational purposes we may define it as a global index of clinical competence in the first year of residency.

Third, the cut-offs used to identify top and bottom groups varied in the different studies. For example, Hojat and colleagues and Markert classified their samples based on the top and bottom 25%; Fincher and colleagues use one-third as the grouping cut-off for top and bottom scorers, and Vu and colleagues used high and low ratings as the criterion measure for grouping their graduates. This lack of unity in group classifications puts certain limitations on combining the data from all medical schools for meta-analytic evaluations. For operational purposes, we define high and low achievers as top and bottom groups, respectively, regardless of the actual cut-off used to determine this typology. In addition, as indicated previously, all data in Table 15.1 are selected for the extreme groups, for example, the top and bottom scorers, excluding the middle groups, with the exception of Vu and colleagues' data, where no middle group was identified. Therefore the combined data in this global analysis have certain limitations. With this in mind, let us examine the data presented in Table 15.1.

A consistent pattern for all the institutions is that the top achievers in medical school are more likely to be rated in the top group in residency (top portion of the table). The reported percentages ranged from 62% for Hojat and colleagues' study to 97% for Fincher and colleagues' study (the lower percentage for the former study could be due to the fact that grades in the first year of medical school were used as the predictor). The figure calculated for the combined data is 75%, indicating that the likelihood of the high achievers in medical school's being rated high on clinical competence in residency is threefold that of their being rated low.

The trend is not as consistent when low achievers in medical school are taken into consideration (bottom portion of the table). The percentages of low achievers in medical school who were also rated in the bottom tail of the competence scale in residency ranged from a high of 76% (Markert's study) to a low of 38% (Vu and colleagues).

The calculated figure for the combined data is 61%, indicating that low achievers in medical school are more than one-and-a-half times as likely to be rated in the bottom as in the top of the competence rating scale in residency. A lack of sharper discrimination in the lower tail of the prediction continuum than in the upper tail can be explained, in part, by the fact that low scorers in medical school, compared with high scorers, are less likely to be represented in the residency assessments, because they either failed in medical school or refused to give permission for their residency evaluations to be studied. The study by Verhulst and Distlehorst in this monograph as well as other studies[13,69] provide support for this proposition. Other factors such as small variability in the entire spectrum of the assessment measures or the presence of differential validity at different levels of the assessment scales can also cast shadows over group distinctions and thus reduce the "hit rate" (see Hojat and colleagues, this monograph) at the bottom tail of the performance measures. The sensitivity and specificity (see Vu and colleagues) of the combined data were .74 and .63, respectively.

To conduct a power analysis and a global meta analytic study of the data reported in Table 15.1, we calculated the chi-square, the coefficient of contingency, the effect size, and the statistical power for each study and for the combined data. The results are presented in Table 15.2.

All chi-square tests were statistically significant at an alpha level of at least .05. The coefficient of contingency is the most widely used measure of association in contingency tables. The values of the effect size (or *W* index; see Cohen[27] [pp. 215–271]) ranged from .24 (for the Vu and colleagues' study) to .49 (for the Markert study). The statistical powers for each study and for the combined data are also reported in the table, with a range from .74 to .99.

Meta-analysis in its conventional sense describes statistical methods for combining the effect sizes of several independent studies using the summary statistics.[125,161] In the present study we used the raw data from five institutions to calculate the combined effect size rather than using the reported statistic for each selected study. The limitations described previously also apply to the combined analysis. The effect size (Cohen's W index) for the combined data, as reported in Table 15.2,

Table 15.2 Inferential and Power Analyses and Effect Sizes of the Selected Data from Empirical Studies Reported in this Monograph and Their Combined Analyses*

Study	Total No of Observations†	Chi-square Value‡	Coefficient of Contingency	Effect Size (*W*)	Statistical Power§
Arnold and Willoughby	66	6.82	.31	.32	.74
Fincher et al.	92	20.10	.42	.47	.99
Hojat et al.	450	29.91	.44	.49	.99
Markert	117	27.87	.44	.49	.99
Vu et al.	133	7.18	.23	.24	.76
Combined data	**858**	**111.33**	**.34**	**.36**	**.99**

*Analyses were performed based on frequency tables of the selected studies presented in Table 1. Combined data are based on cumulative information from the selected studies.

†Total number of observations is based on the frequencies reported in Table 1.

‡All chi-square tests are statistically significant ($p < .05$)

§Statistical power was calculated based on the indicated effect sizes and a probability of type I error (α) equal to .05.

is .36, and the statistical power for the combined data is .99. Cohen[27] (p. 227) describes effect sizes of this magnitude for contingency tables as medium effect sizes. Effect sizes below .30 are considered small and those above .50 are large. Therefore, the values of the effect sizes for individual studies reported in Table 15.2 are mostly in a medium effect-size range, and their statistical powers are generally high. It should be noted that the relatively large sample sizes contribute to these outcomes. Therefore, data reported in Tables 15.1 and 15.2 support the assumption that when considering the high and low achievers in medical school, the competence assessments in residency are significantly associated with those in medical school and a medium effect size is a fair representation of the associations. Reasons for not obtaining a larger effect size are described in our article ("A Case of Mistaken Identity") in this monograph.

In Renschler and Fuchs' study, a sample of German physicians reported that a median of 15% of their knowledge in practice was acquired during medical school training. This area of overlap, when translated into correlation terminology, will be equal to the coefficient of determination, or $r^2 = .15$. The square root of this value ($r = \sqrt{.15} = .39$) will be comparable to the phi coefficients obtained from the data in Table 15.1, which are similar to the effect sizes reported in the Table 15.2. This value is close to the global effect size ($W = .36$) in Table 15.2, indicating that subjective judgments of physicians concerning their applications of knowledge acquired in medical school to practice are consistent with objective indices of overlap between assessments in medical school and in practice.

Our global analysis of the data reported from five medical schools, therefore, supports the proposition that associations between assessments during medical school and ratings of clinical competence in residency exist and are statistically significant. In addition, the statistically significant associations are of practical importance, as indicated by moderate effect sizes obtained. Furthermore, these associations extend beyond residency training, as reported by Case and Swanson and by Hojat and colleagues in this monograph. In both of these studies, failure rates on certifying examinations (Case and Swanson) and board certification status (Hojat and colleagues) were significantly associated with assessments of knowledge in basic sciences made during medical school education. These findings strongly refute the argument of those who propose pessimistically that a good portion of what is learned in medical school is irrelevant to the practice of medicine and therefore must be discarded from the medical school curriculum. What seems irrelevant to them could be of utmost relevance when a decision must be made that could lead to either life or death of a patient (see Vogel, this monograph).

Jensen[83] has claimed that no one has yet been able to devise measures of abilities that do not show positive relationships with one another in a large and representative sample. It has also been suggested that such positive relationships are a result of the general ability, the *sine qua non* of all ability measures, the Spearman's *g* factor.[77,83,170,181] If this assertion is true then are the reported associations attributable to a general ability factor, or the Spearman's *g*, rather than to the genuine relationships between assessments? The fact that conceptually similar measures were associated more strongly than conceptually dissimilar measures (see Hojat and colleagues, and Case and Swanson, this monograph) indicates that sources of variance other than the Spearman's *g* factor contribute to the patterns of the findings. Despite this, untangling the general ability factor from the relationships among assessments in medical school and in practice will be a challenging area for future research.

WHERE DO WE GO FROM HERE?

The contributors to this monograph have produced the most thorough compendium to date of research on the question of the relationship between measures of performance in medical school and in residency. Based on similar longitudinal designs, their work sheds new light on some of the important substantive and methodologic issues that must be addressed in order to understand the connections between medical school and later professional practice. As readers reflect on the papers published here, either to weigh the merits of the individual studies or to plan for the next generation of studies of the connections between medical school and beyond, we recommend that they address the following three questions. First, what is the overall design of the study—how are cohorts tracked and when are performances sampled? Second, what types of instrumentation are used to measure performances in medical school and beyond? And finally, how are the data analyzed and reported? We present an overview of the research presented here, together with our recommendations for further inquiry within these three categories.

Overall Design and Sampling

The value of a longitudinal design to evaluate the connections before and after graduation from medical school is made evident by examining the designs of the empirical studies reported in this monograph.

If we want to serve the public in a better way by assuring that our graduates are competent and capable of rendering the best care, and if we want to evaluate our policies and develop our objectives based on the evolving needs of our society, then we are obligated to monitor our goals, expectations, and outcomes continuously. Longitudinal studies can and do provide critical data needed to evaluate our educational progress and outcomes.

The capacity to document an empirical relationship between medical school and residency is affected first by the overall design of the longitudinal study, in particular the timing of the measurements of performance. The strength of the relationship must be inversely related to the elapsed time between the two measurements, and, as Fincher and colleagues point out, lengthening the time between testings obscures the relationship. In addition, a variety of measurements need to be used both in medical school and during the first year of postgraduate training and afterwards to analyze the relationships.

It is obvious that the most pertinent measurement would be obtained in the early months of the first year of residency, so that the inevitable changes over time would not affect the resident's performance and lessen the empirical relationship with earlier observations made in medical school. Data were obtained near the end of the first year for at least three reasons. First, when global rating scales are used it would be premature for raters to assess residents' performances before having had the opportunity to observe the residents in a variety of clinical situations. Second, the very nature of residency training in the first year involves progressive responsibility for the new residents, and many months are required for the residents to demonstrate their capabilities in a variety of contexts and settings. Finally, from a practical standpoint it would be challenging, at best, to study performance during the summer months of the first year, when new groups of residents are moving into new levels of responsibility. Nevertheless, future studies should be conceptualized so as to minimize the elapsed time between measurements of performances in the two settings.

A second issue related to design and sampling is the effect of the specialty choices of the graduates. In the research of earlier decades, this was inconsequential, since nearly all graduates pursued their first year of training in an undifferentiated program. But now many graduates narrow their specialties early in the first year. The different performances required in different specialties and the varying expectations and standards of performance of different specialties affect the relationship between performances in medical school and in the first postgraduate year.[45,49] It is most likely that the practical constraint of sample size made it impossible for some of the authors to control this effect in the present studies. Further studies need to follow graduates within particular specialty areas.

Similarly, graduates pursue the first year of residency in a variety of settings. The type of hospital—academic medical center, urban public hospital, rural, military, or community hospital—will affect residents' performances. Just as expectations and standards of performance differ among specialties, they also differ among hospitals. Even within the same type of institution, there may be different expectations in ambulatory versus inpatient settings, or different expectations related to new health care delivery systems such as managed care. Although some of the present studies were constrained by sample size, future studies need to be undertaken to control for the variations in performance related to these factors.

The study by Verhulst and colleagues explores an important variation caused by nonresponse bias. While this issue had been given brief attention in many previous follow-up studies of graduates, these researchers attempted to separate the effects of noncompliance of graduates and noncompliance of their program supervisors. It is clear that the bias due to the attrition of graduates with lower levels of performance moderates the empirical link between measures before and after graduation. Further work is needed to develop new methods of increasing the compliance of graduates and their supervisors. Not addressed explicitly in their study, as well as most other published follow-up studies of residents, is the possibility of attrition during the first year of residency. Although low in proportion, some marginal students and residents leave medicine or interrupt their careers; as a result, measurements of their performances cannot be captured in routine follow-up studies.

Finally, it is obvious that other intervening variables will moderate the relationship between medical school and the first year of residency. Vu and colleagues attempted to probe this issue by examining the written comments of graduates whose performances were inconsistent. Perhaps future follow-up studies should explicitly query the supervisors about any personal or other factors that might explain the exemplary or weak performance of a resident.

Multidimensional Measuring Instruments

The complexity of the assessment instruments increases as students advance from medical school to residency and to practice as additional factors play roles in performances beyond medical school.

It is evident that the activities of medical students and the professional tasks of physicians are not equivalent. Medical school students are evaluated largely by their performances on written examinations and to some extent by observations of their clinical skills, assessments of their judgment, and ratings of their clinical competence in controlled situations. Other types of evaluations such as standardized or simulated patients and, recently, computer-based examinations are used to measure students' knowledge and cognitive skills (see McGuire, chapter 1). Data reported by Arnold and Willoughby and by Hojat and colleagues in chapters 7 and 14 indicate that measures of cognitive abilities in medical school are multidimensional. In addition, we proposed that noncognitive measures (personal qualities) also contribute to performances in medical school[70,73,209] (also see McGuire, chapter 1, and "A Case of Mistaken Identity" in chapter 2). The multidimensionality of performance measures in medical school was determined by factor analysis in the studies reported by Arnold and Willoughby and by Hojat and colleagues, which is statistically acceptable, but the resulting dimensions should be conceptually sound.

It should be noted that it may not be enough to factor-analyze several predictor variables and use the resulting common factors as a proxy for a homogeneous predictor variable. This is especially true if the observed scores on the tests comprising a common factor are averaged in an unweighted fashion. The use of weighted factor scores may partially obviate the problem, but missing data may make such an approach unsatisfactory. A factor analysis is capable only of describing the dimensionality of a given set of measures. An obtained structure is therefore subject to considerable change if there is either any variation in the persons providing the data or the addition or deletion of a single variable.

Multidimensional Assessments of Physician Competence

Physicians have many obligations, and to discharge them they must acquire a variety of competencies during medical education and postgraduate training. They are expected to recognize such health-risk factors as hypertension, obesity, and alcoholism and to educate patients as to their implications. In addition, physicians should be able to recognize diseases early,[48] a skill indicative of clinical efficiency. Having recognized a disease or problem, they should treat each patient appropriately, including providing educational support to increase the patient's likelihood of compliance, and should monitor the effectiveness of the treatment. Physicians should also plan for the rehabilitation of a patient if the latter has a chronic health problem and should look for similar health problems in other members of the family and community. These are some of the legitimate responsibilities of physicians that should be learned in medical colleges and afterward. However, all of them can be discharged well without significantly improving the health of patients if the other elements of the health care system are not fulfilling their obligations.

When designing research on the link between medical education and physician performance, it is insufficient to address the simple question: Do good medical students become good doctors? One must identify the components of medical students' competence, namely knowledge, skills, and personal qualities, and study their relationships to corresponding aspects of physicians' competence. A distinction must be made between an individual's acquired knowledge, potential to perform (i.e., his or her competence), and the individual's actual performance. Learning is a necessary but not sufficient condition for performance.[77] Learning provides ingredients for potential performance, and performance requires that the physician go beyond knowledge when performance is demanded and is facilitated by non-physician-related circumstances. It also should be recognized that various factors, only some of which may be under the physician's direct control, impinge upon actual performance. Moreover, competence is itself a complex entity consisting of various components of knowledge, cognitive abilities, psychomotor skills, and personal qualities. Since many different competencies are associated with different medical problems and professional roles, there is a need to develop specific multidimensional instruments that permit performances to be measured in the different areas of interest.

Should such a multidimensional approach not prove feasible in a given situation, we stress that at the very minimum it is important to limit any conclusions based on a piece of the problem under investigation. That is, if we are exploring relationships between information acquired before graduation, we have to caution our readers that a poor resulting correlation says little or nothing about the importance of learning certain information before graduation, for all the many reasons advanced previously. Thus attention must be given to the fact that although the data in this monograph show a relation between what happens in undergraduate medical education and physicians' future performances, intervening variables will confound this relationship. (See chapter 2.) In addition, the effects attributable to specific residency programs need to be taken into consideration. It thus becomes important not only for medical educators to track their graduates in order to evaluate the extent to which desired long-term outcomes are

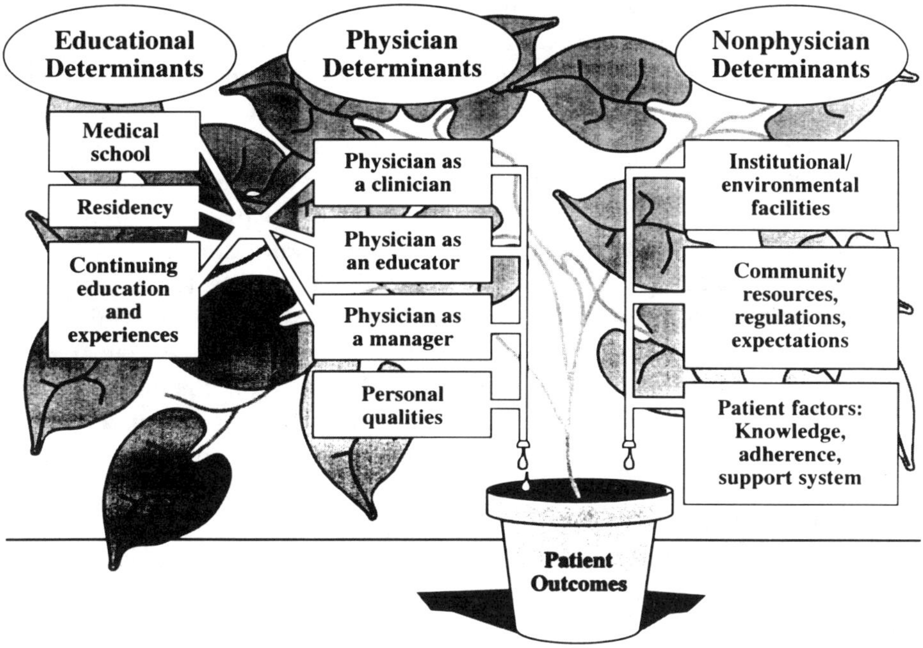

Figure 15.1 Determinants of patient outcomes.

being achieved, but also for the residency programs to do the same thing.

The technology of measuring the knowledge of medical students is more developed than the techniques for assessing skills and attitudes. Measuring patient outcomes and the physician's contribution has improved over the last decade. The measurement of physician performance and resulting inferences regarding competence must take into account variables in career choices and work settings and the contributions of the patients and society. The challenge is how to measure these multidimensional arrays of performances.

Multidimensional Assessments of Components of Patient Care

As depicted in Figure 15.1, three determinants contribute to the outcome of patient care: the educational, physician, and nonphysician determinants. The physician's competence in treating a patient is based on medical knowledge; clinical, pedagogical, and managerial skills acquired in medical school and thereafter; technical abilities; interpersonal skills; and personal qualities.[46,47,50] However, institutional and environmental elements, resources, and expectations, as well as the patient's knowledge, attitudes, and social support system, also affect the quality of the patient's outcome. While the effects of education on the physician's performance are currently a focus of attention, the nonphysician factors, which contribute significantly to outcome measures later in the physician's career, are often ignored or underestimated.

The appropriateness of diagnostic and therapeutic services ordered by physicians is being evaluated by a number of methods. Unfortunately, the methods often fail to distinguish specific skills or behavior that are solely or largely under the control of an individual physician from those that are influenced by nonphysician factors. What is needed is a clear definition of the circumstances under which a measurement should be used and the number of physicians being involved in a particular case. This is especially true when medical record reviews or morbidity data or mortality analysis are done.

Whether some physicians order more diagnostic tests or use more expensive therapeutic agents than others may depend not only on their knowledge or competence but also on other variables such as the severity of the patient's disease,[48] the patient's expectations, the availability of health service resources, and the reward system. As the medical profession and others in society begin to develop methods that measure utilization of resources, careful attention needs to be paid to variables that are not under the control of physicians.

While researchers need to be encouraged to develop new tools, they also need to be required to specify the limitations of their methods. The complexity of measuring the competencies of physicians as clinicians, patient educators, and resource managers needs to be clearly understood when these entities are being assessed using peer ratings, medical record reviews, and morbidity and mortality data. Unless these limitations are made clear, confusion will become greater as to the contribution of the medical school and residency training to the practice of medicine. Measurement of health care results is essential, but the contributions of both physician and nonphysician determinants should be considered.

The contributions of the nonphysician variables produce "noise" that if not controlled becomes louder as the physician advances from residency training to professional practice, hence weakening the associations between medical school and practice performance assessments. We propose that measurement or control of non-physician determinants of patient outcome should be included in the agenda of future research in the assessment of physician performance.

As professional groups, third-party payers, government agencies, and business search for ways to lower health care costs and monitor quality, the use of a variety of medical review methodologies will grow. It is therefore essential that the contributions of physicians or others in the analyses of length of hospital stay, use of diagnostic tests, and mortality reviews be clearly controlled. Even the most competent physician cannot give optimal patient care when practicing in a substandard setting or when the patients are unable or unwilling to assume their share of responsibility for their health care. For instance, some of the variables adversely affecting care are the lack of proper equipment, inadequate personnel support, and a patient population that does not seek medical help early in the course of the disease. Failure to take these into account will result in erroneous conclusions as to the performances and competencies of physicians.

The physician is uniquely responsible for the accuracy of the medical diagnosis and should be able to document and defend the findings reported to a patient. On the other hand, diagnostic efficiency (whether the diagnosis was made early in the evolution of the disease) may be a function of other factors involving the patient and the institution within which care is provided. To analyze accurately the contribution of the physician and to control the influences that the patients, the community, and the institution have on health care, observations should be made prior to, during, and at the end of medical intervention. The severity of the health problems at the time of admission to a hospital or when a patient is first seen by a physician will play a crucial role not only in diagnostic management and subsequent treatment but also in the utilization of health care resources.[48] For instance, the length of stay for a patient who is admitted with appendicitis will depend on whether the appendix is merely inflamed (Stage I), ruptured (Stage II), or ruptured and complicated by systemic infection (Stage III). The medical profession would benefit by classifying health care problems in various severity subgroups in order to measure the various contributions of physicians and those of others in the areas of prevention, diagnostic approach, and therapeutic intervention. The operational scale for determining disease severity is available.[48] Given these issues, assessments and control of the often-ignored area of nonphysician determinants in patient care lay out another challenge for future research.

Multidimensional Assessments of Physician's Roles

We suggest that physicians implicitly play three roles in patient care: *Clinician, patient educator, and resource manager.*[50] Performance in each of these roles is based on knowledge, skills, and personal qualities that can be depicted in a "taxonomy of physician roles and factors in patient care" (see Figure 15.2).

A few examples are given for each cell in the figure. In both the empirical and the nonempirical articles in this monograph, attention is directed almost exclusively to the role of physician as a clinician in the area of knowledge and skills (the two upper-left cells of the taxonomy (Figure 15.2)), while the concepts in the other cells of the figure are largely neglected.

For example, the articles by Nash and colleagues and by Marshall present a multidimensional approach to the assessment of physicians' competencies. While a multidimensional approach must be the method of choice in this kind of assessment, other concepts described in Figure 15.2 should be taken into consideration for a more comprehensive evaluation. Measurement of the concepts in the taxonomy of physician roles and factors in patient outcomes brings yet another challenge for the future research on physician assessments.

The approach most commonly used to evaluate clinical competence has been global rating. The paper by Fincher and colleagues in which supervisors' ratings were compared with graduates' self-ratings reminds us of the inflated and skewed distributions that are commonly reported in global ratings. Unfortunately, published studies have not emphasized interrater reliability and test–retest reliability of the ratings. Nearly all researchers have reported internal consistency estimates of reliability, but these reports tell us little about the critical issues of the perceptions of different raters and their changes over time.

The report of self-ratings (Fincher and colleagues) will remind the reader of other approaches such as peer evaluations that might be used to obtain more valid measurements of residents' performances. As reported by Vu and colleagues, there is increasing interest in the use of standardized patients, and methods such as this or simulated patients may help to control the varying intervening sources for different specialties. Interviewing patients regarding the communication skills of their physician will also provide data to evaluate another important dimension of competence.

Data Analysis

Even after a study has been designed and data have been collected, there are diverse methods of analysis that can be used to estimate the strength of relationships. There now appears to be consensus that correlation coefficients that portray simple linear relationships between medical school and residency are inadequate. While many reports

Physician Factors	Clinician	Patient Educator	Resource Manager
Knowledge	o Knows biophysical and psychosocial factors in disease development o Knows associated risk factors o Knows levels of prevention for stages of disease o Knows appropriate diagnostic and therapeutic procedures	o Knows patient's cultural values and health belief system o Knows level of patient understanding of illness, the rationale for the management plan, expected outcomes and potential economic and social problems o Knows effective methods to modify behavior and enhance compliance	o Knows economic, legal, and ethical ramifications of health behaviors and medical intervention o Knows efficient methods to coordinate care among disciplines o Knows available resources for patient o Knows methods for performing cost-benefit and cost-effective analysis
Skills	o Collects relevant history data o Performs manual skills appropriate to discipline o Interprets lab results appropriately o Makes early and accurate diagnosis o Recognizes risk factors in patient o Develops up-to-date therapeutic and rehabilitation plans o Monitors progress appropriately	o Applies principles of learning and reinforcement o Teaches effectively to assure patient and family understand rationale for management plan, expected outcomes, and potential problems o Encourages compliance with therapeutic plan	o Obtains essential data for decision analysis o Communicates effectively with other members of health care team o Uses human and other resources appropriately o Refers efficiently for consultation diagnostic tests, procedures, and therapeutic intervention
Personal Qualities	o Approaches patient with sensitivity and compassion o Appreciates patient's uniqueness and lifestyle o Adheres to ethical and professional standards	o Considers individual differences in learning styles o Patiently reinforces learning for patient and family	o Facilitates team approach to develop, and implement preventive and therapeutic plan o Involves patient and family in coordinated decisions

Figure 15.2 Physician roles.

have documented stronger relationships at the marginal levels of performance, the opposite trend was found in the studies by Vu and colleagues and by Fincher and colleagues for low scorers in medical school. Future studies with representative samples of residents from the entire range of performance are needed to clarify the predictive relationships.

The studies presented here call attention to the particular problem of establishing standards and cutoffs in order to identify exemplary and marginal residents. Both norm-referenced (where the cutoff is established by examining the performance distribution) and criterion-referenced (where the cutoff is determined by the judgment of experts) cutoffs have been used. Another related assessment issue that contributes not only to the quality of data analysis but also to better identification of marginal performances is the type of measurement scale used. Assessments should be made on a continuous scale rather than a lower type of dichotomous scale (e.g., pass–fail) for better distinction of performances. Those who advocate the pass–fail grading system must realize that assessment is not meant to produce a black-and-white dichotomy. It is also important to identify the gray area in between to locate those who are in need of educational remedies.

One of the critical issues to be addressed in an analysis is the way in which the results and their implications are to be presented to a broad audience. In this regard, the report of Vu and colleagues, in which the framework of sensitivity and specificity is used to describe relationships, deserves special attention. Their nomenclature, which is familiar to clinicians, promises a means of communicating results to a diverse audience of decision makers in medical schools and also allows standardized comparisons of different studies.

At the risk of oversimplification, the one overriding and pervasive weakness that has occurred repeatedly is the failure to ask the right question or to know the real question one is investigating when analyzing a given set of data. Because of the concern and interest in addressing basic issues like quality of care and optimal patient outcomes, investigators are tempted to overgeneralize their findings. Until, for example, we know the contributions of environmental pressures and patient factors to patient outcomes, it is really impossible to relate achievement measures in medical school to measures of patient outcomes and conclude much of anything. A low correlation certainly does not provide evidence that the medical school curriculum is irrelevant to the health of the patient. Thus, eager to improve outcomes, we often jump to conclusions that are unwarranted if we would pause for a moment to think through a logical manner the questions we are really addressing in the data collected and analyzed.

Perhaps the worst mistake is the one some critics are making today. As a result of the inappropriate proposition that a strong relationship between measures before and after graduation does not exist, these critics have mistakenly concluded that medical schools are not doing their jobs. Further, they advocate that changes in the medical curriculum will produce a direct impact on patient outcomes and will solve the deficiencies in the health care system. It may be that the medical school contribution is the easiest to influence, but, if no other message has been conveyed, we hope that this collection of papers helps to clarify that this may be self-delusional. This is not to say that medical education cannot be improved or that more qualified physicians cannot be graduated, but, based on the available evidence and the expanded understanding we trust this document provides, we conclude that we could tinker with the medical school component forever and see little impact on patient outcomes.

To recapitulate, physician competence, physician performance, and appropriate patient care involve a number of complex variables, only some of which can be affected by educational programs. Therefore, above all, let us make sure we are addressing the right question when we analyze the connections between what has been learned in medical school and the performances of physicians in practice. Otherwise, as described in chapter 2 ("A Case of Mistaken Identity"), the contaminating factors will produce "noise" that obscures the strength of the "signal" even more seriously when coupled with our ignorance. The complexity of assessments and their pertinent issues may raise more questions than answers. We believe that awareness of the pertinent issues can lead to better-stated questions and better-formulated hypotheses. A question well-stated is a question half answered, and a hypothesis well-formulated is a hypothesis half tested. We hope that this monograph will redirect and shorten the path to understanding the complexity of assessments in medical school, in practice, and in patient outcomes and will make future research more fruitful. We have a long way to go—we hope that this publication paves the road for fruitful explorations.

CHAPTER SIXTEEN

International Perspectives

Bingxun Liu, M.D.,
Charles Boelen, M.D., D.P.H., M.Sc.,
David M. Macfadyen, M.B.ch.B., F.R.C.P., Edin., and
Horacio J. A. Rimoldi, M.D., Ph.D.

Dispelling the Myth

Bingxun Liu, M.D.

The contribution of this monograph by the editors and their collaborators will be invaluable to the field of medical education. The association between measures of academic performances in medical school and performances in practice has been an important theoretical and practical issue and a topic of enduring interest for medical educators all over the world for a very long time. As mentioned by the editors of the monograph, the issue had long been debated but was not settled because previous findings seemed inconsistent. The issue is settled now because the monograph provides consistent evidence in support of the proposition that performances in medical school have relevance to those in practice.

Professional education can be aimless if the assumption raised by the editors ("A Case of Mistaken Identity") on the continuity from one level of training to another is not supported. The issue of continuity at internship training has also been addressed in the People's Republic of China by collecting data on residents. The continuity assumption was supported by resulting associations between scores on the Chinese National Medical Examination (taken at the end of the first year of residency) and clinical competence ratings by program directors two years later.[212] As described in this monograph (see "A Case of Mistaken Identity,"and "Is the Glass Half Full or Half Empty,"), specialty areas were also found to contribute to the strength of the association in our study in China, which suggest that the "noise" which obscures the "signal" can be equally applicable to the data from other countries regardless of geographical boundaries.

This monograph is a landmark document that dispels the myth that no meaningful continuity or association should be expected between performance measures throughout medical training and practice.

Opening of a Promising Area of Investigation

Charles Boelen, M.D., D.P.H., M.Sc.

Rigorous approaches to assessing and justifying the way doctors are educated are needed but are not yet common. As such approaches become better developed and known, their use will logically take precedence over the use of subjective criteria such as common sense, consensus among peers, individual or group experience, and sometimes fashion or imitation.

We often hear: "This school is known to be good for (community medicine, thoracic surgery, obstetrics and gynecology, etc.)." Such statements are not uncommonly made by senior staff members themselves about the quality of the educational institutions they run. Reputations for excellence can arise in this way and may remain uncontested due to lack of objective and valid yardsticks. In the case of medical education, it is appalling to note that so many judgments and decisions for action are being made without objective support by otherwise distinguished scientists. In the reform of medical education, subjectivity has too often been the rule, and objectivity the exception.

Education in general, with its link to the sociocultural context, is still widely considered a soft science and therefore governed more often by opinions than by hard facts. This may explain the widespread tendency to treat lightly the fate of medical education. With the advent of assessment measures, promoters of medical education reforms by intuitive means will progressively give way to new leaders guided by research findings.

This book sheds light on the purpose and modalities of the search for evidence of the validity of the medical educational process. Creative thinking and persistent research will eventually produce the proven methodologies and objective measurement tools that are essential to connect performance in medical schools with outcome in medical practice and health care. As a consequence, medical education will gain respectability as a scientific discipline; verification of the impact of education on health care will be spurred; understanding between health policy makers, academic institutions and the medical profession will be improved; and international collaboration will be enhanced.

We may all have heard of health statistics showing that health indicators in a given country or region had improved while doctors were on strike or when the doctor/population ratio had decreased. Such instances illustrate the ambiguity that the medical profession faces. On one hand, physicians are seen as driving the health system—although nowadays, increasingly, the contrary may be true. On the other hand, due to the many factors influencing health, a growing number of which are from outside the health sector, it is difficult to demonstrate or to refute the specific impact of doctors' performance on health status.

Poorly substantiated correlation causes malaise that only a dispassionate and objective approach can alleviate. Standardized definitions are required to delineate the functions of a doctor, to specify the nature and quality of services rendered, and to describe the circumstances under which these services are rendered. And medical schools will have to determine how they can optimally respond.

Besides the usual diagnostic and therapeutic skills, there is a surprisingly unanimous call worldwide for doctors possessing aptitudes in the promotion of healthy lifestyles, the appropriate selection and use of technologies—from the point of view not only of efficacy but also of economy and of ethics—and the improvement of quality of care, taking into account individual needs and the needs of society at large. To become accountable to society for the quality of graduates and their capacity to apply skills for the benefit of people's health, medical schools should accept and be able to assume new responsibilities outside of their usual realm, namely in preparing the working environment of their future graduates. Their active involvement in health services research, in testing alternative practice patterns, and in ensuring quality in health care will indeed help create a climate in which clearer connections between the education of doctors and their professional performance can be established.

The assumption prevails that excellence in the learning process determines the quality of graduates, and, by extension, the quality of professional performance. This assumption is now being questioned, however, as the need for cost-effectiveness is more widely felt. The interest we are now witnessing in assessing a medical school's performance demonstrates how far and fast ideas may evolve. Medical education will be viewed in a perspective not limited to curricular innovations, and the impact of education on medical practice and health care will be more widely studied.

The merit of the authors is to imply that if the search for objectivity is maintained, the drive to link medical education with medical practice will lead medical education to extend its responsibility beyond curriculum development. By courageously exposing itself to scrutiny by outcome measures, medical education will acquire a social and political dimension, and medical schools may become better recognized as valid partners in health care organization and management issues important for their local communities and the nation as a whole.

As a natural flow from quality medical education to quality medical care needs to be established, the challenge of setting standards that will eventually allow the measurement of quality in medical care and in medical education will foster the creation of new alliances between the medical school and the health sector. The study of correlation between student performance and excellence in professional practice opens the way for a basic interrogation of the capacity of a medical school to respond to society's health needs, since reflection on educational outcomes cannot be isolated from reflection on outcomes of medical school interventions in research and in health service delivery. Thus, in systematically examining the relevance of education, medical schools should be led also to assess the relevance to and impact of their research and health service activities on health care.

The myth of international standards in medical education is far from being dispelled, as may be noted from brochures promoting educational programs, for example. We should, however, clearly distinguish the goal of establishing standards of universal value from the establishment of international standards. While a worldwide uniform medical curriculum disregarding specific needs of the cultural, epidemiological, and socioeconomic context is to be avoided, a global consensus is desirable and possible on essential functions of a physician, on essential features of the mission of a medical school, and on essential characteristics of a medical education program, as well as on the necessity for constant adaptation to a changing environment. Of course, to fully ensure social relevance, the objectives of a health system, expressed through national health policies and health priorities, should remain the ultimate reference.

With the accelerating rate of global information flow and the increasing mobility of the medical profession, institutions and countries are rapidly becoming more interested in defining quality in medical education, in terms of both process and outcome, that would be accepted worldwide. If carefully designed and constantly improved through research, indicators of quality are likely to be welcomed by the academic community.

Universally recognized yardsticks would give health leaders and medical educators in many countries the confidence to plan and organize the education of their physicians in an unbiased manner, liberating themselves from foreign models that do not always fit the requirements of their environment.

It will be a long march before objective measurement tools are available and widely recognized and applied to guide the education of doctors, but on the whole, the sentiment of the "glass half-full" expressed by the authors appropriately reflects the opening of a promising area of investigation.

An Affirmative Answer to the Key Question

David M. Macfadyen, M.B.ch.B., F.R.C.P., Edin.

Separating "signal" from "noise" is an apt analogy for this major review of global efforts to predict the outcome of medical education. The "noise" which blocks out a clear perception of the signal (see chapter 2) emanates from a preoccupation with the technology of educational measurement, which is understandable in view of the very great volume of data collected. However a clear signal beams through this vast data because, at the outset, the editors posed the following simple question: Are low and high standings in medical school significantly associated with corresponding standings in clinical competence ratings in residency? This leads this writer to the conclusion that the end point of educational measurement in medical school is to detect correctly high performance in residency and not to miss low performance in residency. Noise might be minimized and clarity increased by concentrating on analytic methods that generate such *discrimination* in measured residency performance from the whole array of measurements made during medical education. Moreover, the language of discrimination ("hits" and "misses" in the article by Hojat and colleagues or "sensitivity" and "specificity" in the article by Vu and colleagues) presents educational measurement in terms that faculty members and students can easily comprehend.

Longitudinal studies in medical education generate an array of measurements during the whole period of medical education—more robust in the preclinical years when the building blocks for future learning are laid. This array of measures can be used singly or in aggregate to predict good and poor performance during residency (and, by extrapolation, in medical practice). An ultimate point against which the process of medical education might be measured is an aggregate score generated from a consistent set of items on a standard resident supervisor's rating form.

In their conclusions (chapter 15) the editors are correct in drawing special attention to the framework for sensitivity and specificity to describe these relationships. As illustrated in Tables 15.1 and 15.2 of chapter 15, this framework has allowed comparison between different longitudinal studies. It has also allowed the results of different studies to be combined in a "meta-analysis" described in chapter 15. Thus the key question asked by the editors is answered in the affirmative and, in the process of doing so, they have brought greater clarity to the analyses of present and future longitudinal assessments of the outcome of medical education.

Assessments in Medical Education: Looking Beyond a Point of No Return

Horacio J. A. Rimoldi, M.D., Ph.D.

Inspection of the published books and articles related to the subject discussed in this monograph shows that from a few studies published around 1950, the number has increased considerably since the 1970s. This points to the development of a relatively new field of research with wide theoretical implications that reach the field of education, diagnosis, treatment, follow up of patients, continued education, organization of health services and more recently, the cost of medical services that originated the concept of "staging" as developed by J. Gonnella and Associates.

Indeed, the quantity and quality of reports ranging from those which are excellent to those of questionable merit make it difficult to reach a fair overall judgment. It should be added that the appropriateness of the kind of methods employed amounts, in some cases, to a questionable use of powerful techniques not necessarily justified. As B. Shaw[213] masterly stated, "the test of sanity is not the normality of the method but the reasonableness of the discovery." The last test resides in reaching the kind of closure that as H. Poincare[214] demanded generalizes the diversity into a comprehensive unity. The authors of this monograph have done this, synthesizing a vast amount of data into a few well-established, reliable and valid statements that transcend specificities; exemplifying what can be done when careful analysis and scientific equanimity are the means used to better understand.

This monograph is a landmark in the history of assessment of medical performance at different levels of sophistication, and as it should be, the underlying plan seems to be based on the idea that the progress of science requires the sequential process that transform some of day-today orthodoxies into heterodoxies that tomorrow may in turn become new orthodoxies. And so, the sequence goes on endlessly.

Reaching a new goal opens new views and these demand new ways to find out what it all means. This monograph is "a point of no return" by pointing to those interested in medical education: a) paths to be traveled in the future, b) paths that have become landmarks not to be ignored, and c) paths that have shown to be worthless. All this could be summarized by saying that this monograph represents a major future research project that awaits implementation.

The four investigators who have written and selected the significant studies assembled in this monograph form a well-organized team of medical educators who have contributed across the years to improve assessment, to invent procedures to do so, to critically examine their own efforts, and to join theory and practice, blending hypotheses and facts. What they present works because it is true to the facts, and it is sound because it is true to logic.

The monograph begins with a historical presentation of the problems that have concerned those interested in the teaching of medicine. This is followed by some selected studies conducted by investigators from different schools, and the presentation is crowned with the editors' conclusions that are aptly stated by asking: "What have we learned, and where do we go from here?"—after asking paradoxically: "Is the glass half full or half empty?"—and, I say paradoxically, because their presentation fills the glass from which many have drunk.

In this meta-analytic study the conclusion about the associations between performances in medical school and after graduation, the specificity of these associations depending on specialization, and the influence of personality measures are highlighted. Their findings "indicate that significant associations exist among . . . performance measures in medical school and ratings of postgraduate competence in data-gathering and processing skills," that "the strengths of the associations varied for different areas of postgraduate competence," and that stronger associations appear between "global assessments of clinical competence in medical school and assessment of postgraduate clinical competence" when conceptually similar measures are explored.

The contributors to this publication are known investigators working in different U.S. universities; interested in problems of assessment of medical competence and on the teaching of medicine. However, the problems they discuss and most of the solutions and conclusions reached have clear application in the area of medical education throughout. Thus, beyond the local characteristics that a given problem may have, many of their conclusions go beyond localisms and may be widely applied regardless of the specificity of the situation under which they were examined. Thus it is for the intelligent reader to examine critically how and which of the obtained results help to clarify and solve the problems he or she has to face in different environments. The instructor can then use this information to generalize and solve problems beyond the limits of the specific event.

These findings refute the pessimistic view which claims that what is learned in "medical school is irrelevant to the practice of medicine" thus settling a long overdue controversy. A new field has been opened when "learning is a necessary but not sufficient condition for performance." We may add that by implying that knowledge is different from understanding, future research efforts should aim to explore how, when and which are the elements necessary to succeed in the performance of medical tasks. That is, in which way should we ask; when, that is, in which sequence should we ask and; which, that is, what are the things we should ask? Old fashioned testing techniques should be complemented by new approaches that should include the sequential processing of data, subsequent or concomitant to information gathering, in order to attempt to reach a conclusion that goes beyond what is already known. This is implied throughout this monograph.

In short, the progress of knowledge brings change, including the discovery of new paths and the closing of others. This implies learning to learn and learning to "unlearn" so that new vistas may either replace or reaffirm old ones. Unless we prefer to assume that going round in circles is equivalent to moving forward, as Lewis Carroll so aptly wrote: "Now, here you see, it takes all the running you can do, to keep in the same place."[215]

References

1. Abrahamson, S. Report to the Royal Australian College of General Practitioners. Unpublished. Melbourne, Australia, 1987.
2. Abrahamson, S. Offices of Research in Medical Education: "What Have You Guys Ever Done Anyway?" *Acad. Med.* **66**, Supp. (Sept. 1991):S89–S92.
3. Ackerman, F.K., and Nash, D.B. Teaching the Tenets of Quality: A Survey of Medical Schools and Programs in Health Administration. *Qual. Rev. Bull.* **17** (1991):200–203.
4. Aiken, L.R. The Problem of Nonresponse in Survey Research. *J. Experimental Educ.* **56** (1988):116–119.
5. Albo, D.Jr., Taylor, C.W., & Page, B. Evaluating the Performance of Resident Physicians Against the Target of Excellent Physicians-in-Practice. In *Evaluation of Non-Cognitive Skills and Clinical Performance*, J.S. Lloyd ed., pp. 113–126. Chicago, IL: American Board of Medical Specialists.
6. American College of Physicians. *Hospital Clinical Privileges Guidelines for Procedures in Gastroenterology and Nephrology.* Philadelphia, PA: Clinical Privileges Project, American College of Physicians, 1990.
7. American Medical Review Research Center (AMRRC). A Proposal to Develop, Apply and Evaluate Review Criteria and Educational Outreach Programs Based Upon Practice Guidelines. RFP#282-91-0074, The Agency for Health Care Policy and Research, Washington, DC August 28, 1991.
8. Arnold, L. Willoughby, T.L., & Calkins, E.V. Understanding the Clinical Competence of Physicians: A Factor Analysis Approach. *J. Med. Educ.* **59** (1984):591–594.
9. Arnold, L., Willoughby, T.L., & Calkins, E.V. Self-Evaluation in Undergraduate Medical Education: A Longitudinal Perspective. *J. Med. Educ.* **60** (1985):21–28.
10. Association of American Medical Colleges. Physicians for the Twenty-First Century: Report of the Project Panel on the General Professional Education of the Physician. *J. Med. Educ.* **59** Part 2 (1984).
11. Barrows, H.S. *Simulated (Standardized) Patients and Other Human*

Stimulations. Chapel Hill, NC: Health Sciences Consortium, 1987.

12. Blacklow, R.S., Goepp, C.E., & Hojat, M. Class Ranking Models for Dean's Letters and Their Psychometric Evaluation. *Proc. Ann. Conf. Res. Med. Educ.* In *Acad. Med.* **66**, Supp. (September 1991): S10–S12.
13. Blacklow, R.S., Goepp, C.E., & Hojat, M. Further Psychometric Evaluations of A Class Ranking Model as a Predictor of Graduate' Clinical Competence in the First Year of Residency. *Acad. Med.*, in press, April, 1993.
14. Bloom, B.S. (Ed) *Taxonomy of Educational Objectives*—The Classification of Educational Goals. Handbook 1: The Cognitive Domain. New York: Longman Green, 1965.
15. Bloom, S.W. The Medical School as a Social Organization: The Sources of Resistance to Change. *Med. Educ.* **23** (1989):228–241.
16. Bott, E.A. The Predictive Value of College Marks in Medical Subjects. *J. Med. Res.*, **12** (1925):214–227.
17. Bourne, L.E., & Ekstrand, B.R. *Psychology: Its Principles and Meaning*. Hinsdale, IL: Dryden, 1973.
18. Brennan, T.A., Leape, L.L., Laird, N.M., Herbert, L., Localio, A.R., Lawthers, A.G., Newhouse, J.P., Weiler, P.C., & Hiatt, H.H. Incidence of Adverse Events and Negligence in Hospitalized Patients. Results of the Harvard Medical Practice Study I. *N. Engl. J. Med.* **324** (1991):370–376.
19. Bull, G.M. An Examination of the Final Examination in Medicine. *Lancet* **2** (1956):368–372.
20. Calhoun, J.G., Wolf, F.M., Maxim, B.R., & Davis, W.K. Validity Coefficients of Clinical Competence on NBME Part III Examinations. *J. Med. Educ.* **60** (1985):189–192.
21. Calhoun, J.G., Wooliscroft, J.O., TenHaken, J.D., Wolf, F.M., & Davis, W.K. Evaluating Medical Student Clinical Skill Performance: Relationships Among Self, Peer, and Expert Ratings. *Eval. Health Prof.* **11** (1988):201–212.
22. Campbell, D.T., & Fiske, D.W. Convergent and Discriminant Validation by the Multitrait-Multimethod Matrix. *Psychol. Bull.* **56** (1959):81–105.
23. Carrol, J.B. The Nature of Data, or How to Choose a Correlation Coefficient. *Psychometrika* **26** (1961):347–372.
24. Catalano, R.A., & Jenkins, P.L. Correlating Factors to Resident performance in an Opthalmology Program. *Opthalmology* **96** (1989): 552–554.
25. Clute, K.F. *The General Practitioner: A Study of Medical Education and Practice in Ontario and Nova Scotia*. Toronto: University of Toronto Press, 1963.
26. Clyman, S.G., & Orr, N.A. Status Report on the NBME's Computer-based Testing. *Acad. Med.* **65** (1990):235–241.

27. Cohen, J. *Statistical Power Analysis for the Behavioral Sciences*. Hillsdale, NJ: Lawrence Erlbaum, 1987.
28. Curry, R.H., Yarnold, P.R., Bryant, F.B., Martin, G.J., & Hughes, R. L. A Path Analysis of Medical School and Residency Performance: Implications for Housestaff Selection. *Eval. Health Prof.* **11** (1988): 113–129.
29. Darlington, R.B. Multiple Regression in Psychological Research and Practice. *Psychol. Bull.* **69** (1968):161-182.
30. Dinham, S.M. & Barbee, R.A. Assessment of Three-year Versus Four-year Medical School Graduates. *Eval. Health Prof.* **1** (1978):25–34.
31. Distlehorst, L.H., Verhulst, S.J., Vu, N.V., & Barrows, M.D. The Use of Performance-Based Assessment Scores and Traditional Measures in Predicting First-Year Residency Performance. *Proc. Annu. Conf. Res. Med. Educ.* **27** (1988):176–181.
32. Donabedian, A. The Epidemiology of Quality. *Inquiry* **22** (1985): 176–181.
33. Dowaliby, F.J., & Andrew, B.J. Relation Between Clinical Competence Ratings and Examination Performance. *J. Med. Educ.* **51** (1976):181–188.
34. Edinburgh Declaration. Edinburgh, Scotland: World Federation for Medical Education, 1988.
35. Erlandson, E.E., Calhoun, J.G., Barrack, F.M., Hull, A.L., Youmans, L.C., Davis, W.K., & Bartlett, R.H. Resident Selection: Applicant Selection Criteria Compared with Performance. *Surgery.* **92** (1982):270–275.
36. Fabb, W.E., & Marshall, J.R. *The Assessment of Clinical Competence*: Lancaster, England; Boston, MA; The Hague, The Netherlands: MTP Press, 1983.
37. Flood, A.B., Scott, W.R., Ewy, W., & Forrest, W.H. Effectiveness in Professional Organizations: The Impacts of Surgeons and Surgical Staff Organization on the Quality of Care in Hospitals. *Health. Serv. Res.* **17** (1982):341–366.
38. Freund, R.F., & Minton, P.D. *Regression Methods*. New York: Marcel Dekker, 1979.
39. Fricke, B.G. Review of the College Entrance Examination Board Admission Testing Program. In *The Sixth Mental Measurements Yearbooks*, O.K. Buros, Ed., pp. 975–988. Highland Park, NJ: Gryphos Press, 1965.
40. Gaier, E.L. The Criterion Problem in the Prediction of Medical School Success. *J. Appl. Psychol.* **36** (9152):316–322.
41. George, J.M., Young, D., & Metz, E.N. Evaluating Selected Internship Candidates and Their Subsequent Performances. *Acad. Med.* **64** (1989):480–482.
42. Ghiselli, E.E. The Validity of Aptitude Tests in Personnel Selection.

Personnel Psychol. **26** (1973):461–477.

43. Glass, G.V., & Stanley, J.C. *Statistical Methods in Education and Psychology*, Englewood Cliffs, NJ: Prentice-Hall, 1970.
44. Goldman, R.L. The Reliability of Peer Assessments of Quality of Care. *JAMA* **267** (1992):958–960.
45. Gonnella, J.S. & Hojat, M. Relationship Between Performance in Medical School and Postgraduate Competence. *J. Med. Educ.* **58** (1983):679–685.
46. Gonnella, J.S., Hojat, M., Veloski, J.J., and Zeleznik, C. Measuring the Contribution of Medical Education to Patient Care: A Review. In *Research in Medical Education: 1983. Proceedings of the Twenty-second Annual Conference.* S. Kerby, Compiler, pp. 3–16. Washington, DC: Association of American Medical Colleges, 1983.
47. Gonnella, J.S., Hojat, M., Veloski, J.J., & Zeleznik, C. Competence Assessment During Medical School. In *Proceedings of Conference on Physician Competence: Whose Responsibility.* I. Singer, Ed., pp. 53–62. Houston, TX: American Medical Association, American Hospital Association, and Association of American Medical Colleges, 1988.
48. Gonnella, J.S., Hornbrook, M.C., & Louis, D.Z. Staging of Disease: A case-mix Measurement. *JAMA*, **251** (9184):637–644.
49. Gonnella, J.S., & Veloski, J.J. The Impact of Early Specialization on the Clinical Competence of Residents. *N. Engl. J. Med.* **306** (1982):275–277.
50. Gonnella, J.S., Veloski, J.J., Xu, G., & Hojat, M. The Challenges in Measuring Educational Outcomes. Paper presented at the 50th Anniversary Conference of the Liaison Committee on Medical Education. Chicago, IL, 1992.
51. Gordon, R.A. Issues in Multiple Regression. *Am. J. Sociology,* **73** (1968):592–616.
52. Gough, H.G., & Hall, W.B. An Attempt to Predict Graduation from Medical School. *J. Med. Educ.* **50** (1975):940–950.
53. Gough, H.G., & Hall, W.B. The Prediction of Academic and Clinical Performance in Medical School. *Res. Higher Educ.* **3** (1975): 301–314.
54. Gough, H.G., Hall, W.B., & Harris, R.E. Evaluation of Performance in Medical Training. *J. Med. Educ.* **39** (1964):679–692.
55. Grand'Maison, P., Lescop, J., Rainsberry, P., & Brailovsky, C.A. Large Scale Use of An Objective, Structured Clinical Examination for Licensing Family Physicians. *Can. Med. Assoc. J.* **146** (192): 1735–1740.
56. Grant, J., & Marsden, P. The Structure of Memorized Knowledge in Students and Clinicians: An Explanation for Diagnostic Expertise. *Med. Educ.* **21** (1987):92–98.
57. Grant, J., & Marsden, P. Primary Knowledge, Medical Education and Consultant Expertise. *Med. Educ.* **22** (1988):173–179.

58. Guadagnoli, E., and Cunningham S. The Effects of Nonresponse and Late Response on a Survey of Physician Attitudes. *Eval. Health Prof.* **12** (1989):318–328.
59. Guilford, J.P. *Fundamental Statistics in Psychology and Education*. NY: McGraw-Hill, 1965.
60. Gunzberger, L.K., Frazier, R.G., Yang, L.M., Rainey, M.L., & Wronski, T. Premedical and Medical School Performance in Predicting First-year Residency Performance. *J. Med. Educ.* **62** (1987):379–384.
61. Harden, R.M., & Gleeson, F.A. Assessment of Clinical Competence Using an Objective Structured Clinical Examination (OSCE). Medical Education Booklet No. 8. Dundee, Scotland: Association for the Study of Medical Education, 1979.
62. Hart, I.R., & Harden, R.M. *Further Developments in Assessing Clinical Competence*. International Conference Proceedings. Montreal, PQ: Can-Heal Publications, 1987.
63. Hart, I.R., Harden, R.M., & Walton, H.J., Eds. *Newer Developments in Assessing Clinical Competence*. International Conference Proceedings. Montreal, PQ: Can-Heal Publications, 1986.
64. Henbest, R.J., & Fehrsen, G.S. Preliminary Study at the medical University of Southern Africa on Student Self-Assessment as a Means of Evaluation. *J. Med. Educ.* **60** (1985):66–68.
65. Herman, H.H. *Modern Factor Analysis*. (rev. ed.) Chicago, IL: The University of Chicago Press, 1976.
66. Herman, M.W., Veloski, J. & Hojat, M. Validity and Importance of Low Ratings Given to Medical School Graduates in Noncognitive Areas. *J. Med. Educ.* **58** (1983):837–843.
67. Hildreth, E.A. A New Look at Clinical Privileges for Procedures. *Ann. Intern. Med.* **107** (1987):585–587.
68. Hojat, M., Borenstein, B.D., & Veloski, J.J. Cognitive and Noncognitive Factors in Predicting the Clinical Performance of Medical School Graduates. *J. Med. Educ.* **63** (1988):323–325.
69. Hojat, M., Gonnella, J.S., & Veloski, J.J. Performance in medical School and Postgraduate Clinical Competence: An Empirical Study of Methodological and Conceptual Issues. Paper presented at the Annual Meeting of the American Educational Research Association, San Francisco, CA, April, 1986.
70. Hojat, M., Robeson, M., Damjanov, I., Veloski, J.J., & Zeleznik, C. Performance in Medical School as a Function of Psychosocial Characteristics. Paper presented at the Centennial Convention of the American Psychological Association, Washington, DC, August 1992.
71. Hojat, M., & Veloski, J.J. Subtest Scores of a Comprehensive Examination of Medical Knowledge as a Function of Retention Interval. *Psychol. Rep.* **55** (1984):579–586.

72. Hojat, M., Veloski, J.J., & Borenstein, B.D. Components of Clinical Competence Ratings: An Empirical Approach. *Educ. Psychol. Meas.* **46** (1986):761–769.
73. Hojat, M., Vogel, W.H., Zeleznik, C., & Borenstein, B.D. Effects of Academic and Psychosocial Predictors of Performance in medical School on Coefficients of Determinations. *Psychol. Rep.* **63** (1988): 383–394.
74. Hubbard, J.P., & Clemans, W.V. *Multiple Choice Examinations in Medicine: A Guide for Examiner and Examinee.* Philadelphia, PA: Lea and Febiger, 1961.
75. Huebner, L.A., Roger, J.A., & Moore, J. The Assessment and Remediation of Dysfunctional Stress in Medical School. *J. Med. Educ.* **56** (1981):547–558.
76. Hunt, D.D., Scott, C.S., Phillips, T.J., Yergan, J., & Greig, L.M. Performance of Residents Who Had Academic Difficulties in Medical School. *J. Med. Educ.* **62** (1987):170–179.
77. Hunter, J.E. Cognitive Ability, Cognitive Aptitude, Job Knowledge, and Job Performance. *J. Vocational Behav.* **29** (1986):340–362.
78. Iezzoni, L.I. "Black Box" Medical Information Systems: A Technology Needing Assessment. *JAMA* **265** (1991):3066–3067.
79. Iglehart, J.K. Germany's Health Care System. *N. Engl. J. Med.* **324** (1991):1750–1756.
80. Iglehart, J.K. Germany's Health Care System (Second of Two Parts). *N. Engl. J. Med.* **324** (1991):1750–1756.
81. Jacobsen, T.L., Price, P.B., DeMilk, G.H., & Taylor, C.W. *An Exploratory Study of Predictors of Physician Performance.* Cooperative Research Program Contract No. OE-3-10-136. Washington, DC: U.S. Department of Health, Education and Welfare, 1965.
82. Jencks, S.F., & Wilensky, G.R. The Health Quality Improvement Initiative: A New Approach to Quality Assurance in Medicare. *JAMA* **268** (1992):900–903.
83. Jensen, A.R. G: Artifact or Reality. *J. Vocational Behav.* **29** (1986): 301–331.
84. Johnson, V., Miller, R.D., & Gage, R.D. Correlation Between Performance in medical School and in Residency Training. *J. Med. Educ.* **38** (1963):591–595.
85. Kaiser, H. The Application of Electronic Computers to Factor Analysis. *Educ. Psychol. Meas.* **20** (1960):141–151.
86. Kane, M.T. The Assessment of Professional Competence. *Eval. Health Prof.* **15** (1992):163–182.
87. Kasper, J.F., Plume, S.K., & O'Connor, G.T. A Methodology for QI in the Coronary Artery Bypass Grafting Procedure Involving Comparative Analysis. *Qual. Rev. Bull.* **18** (1992):129–133.
88. Kassebaum, D.G. The Measurement of Outcomes in the Assessment

of Educational Program Effectiveness. *Acad. Med.* **65** (1990):293–296.

89. Keck, J.S., Arnold, L., Willoughby, L., & Calkins, V. Efficacy of Cognitive/Noncognitive Measures in Predicting Resident-Physician Performance. *J. Med. Educ.* **54** (1979):759–765.
90. Kegel-Flom, P. Predicting Supervisor, Peer, and Self Ratings of Intern Performance. *J. Med. Educ.* **50** (1975):812–815.
91. Kellie, S.E., & Kelly, J.T. Medicare Peer Review Organization Preprocedure Review Criteria: An Analysis of Criteria for Three Procedures. *JAMA* **265** (1991):1265–1270.
92. Kidder, I.H. & Judd, C.M. Research methods in Social Relations. (5th ed.) Published for the Society for the Psychological Study of Social Issues (SPSSI). New York: Holt, Rinehart and Winston, 1986.
93. Klatzky, R.L. *Human Memory: Structure and Process.* (2nd ed.) San Francisco: Freeman, 1975.
94. Kolm, P. & Verhulst, S.J. Comparing Self- and Supervisor Evaluations. *Eval. Health Prof.* **10** (1987):80–89.
95. Korman, M., & Stubblefield, R.L. Medical School Evaluation and Internship Performance. *J. Med. Educ.* **46** (1971):670–673.
96. Krathwohl, D.R., Bloom, B.S., & Masia, B.B. *Taxonomy of Educational Objectives—The Classification of Educational Goals. Handbook 1: The Affective Domain.* New York: Longman Green, 1965.
97. Kroenke, K. Attending Rounds: Guidelines for Teaching on the Wards. *J. Gen. Int. Med.* **7** (1992):68–75.
98. Kron, I.L., Kaiser, D.L., Nolan, S.P., Rudolf, L.E., Muller, W.H., & Jones, R.S. Can Success in the Surgical Residency Be Predicted from Pre-Residency Evaluation? *Ann. Surg.* **202** (1985):694–695.
99. Kumpusalo, E., Mattila, K., Virjo, I., Neittaanmaki, L., Kataja, V., Jujala, S., Jaaskelainen, M., Luhtata, R., & Isokoski, M. Medical Education and the Corresponding Professional Needs of Young Doctors: The Finnish Junior Physician 88 Study. *Med. Educ.* **25** (1991):71–77.
100. Kupfer, D.J., Drew, F.L., Curtis, E.K., & Rubinstein, D.N. Personality Style and Empathy in Medical Students. *J. Med. Educ.* **53** (1978): 507–509.
101. Langsley, D.G. Medical Competence and Performance Assessment. A New Era. *JAMA* **266** (1991):977–980.
102. Last, J.M., Martin, F.M., & Stanley, G.R. Academic Record and Subsequent career. *Proc. R. Soc. Med.* **60** 91967):813–816.
103. Lau, A.W., Taylor, C.W., Nelson, D.E., & Price, P.B. Relationship of Premedical and Medical Grades to Physician Performance measures. Paper presented at the Rocky Mountain Psychological Association annual convention, Phoenix, AZ, 1975.
104. Lawthers, A.G. Center for Research on Health Care Quality, Har-

vard University, Cambridge, Massachusetts. Personal communication, March 31, 1992.

105. Leape, L.L., Brennan, T.A., Laird, N., Lawthers, A.G., Localio, A.R., Barnes, B.A., Herbert, L., Newhouse, M.P., Weiler, P.C., & Hiatt, H. The Nature of Adverse Events in Hospitalized Patients. *N. Engl. J. Med.* **324** (1991):377–384.

106. Levine, H.G., Yunker, R., & Bec, D. Pediatric Resident Performance: The Reliability and Validity of Rating Forms. *Eval. Health. Prof.* **9** (1986):62–74.

107. Levinson, D.J. Medical Education and the Theory of Adult Socialization. *J. Health Soc. Behav.* **8** (1967):253–265.

108. Linn, B.S., & Zeppa, R. Stress in Junior Medical Students Relationships to Personality and Performance. *J. Med. Educ.* **59** (1984):7–12.

109. Lockyer, J.M. Physician Performance: The Roles of Knowledge, Skill, and Environment. *Teach. Learn. Med.* **4** (1992):86–96.

110. Loftus, L.S., Arnold, L., & Willoughby, T.L. First-year Residents' Performances Compared with Their Medical School Class Ranks as Determined by Three Ranking Systems. *Acad. Med.* **67** (1992): 319–323.

111. Mackowiak, R., & Gonnella, J.S. Clinical Competence as measured by the national Boards, Part III. *Proc. Annu. Conf. Res. Med. Educ.* **12** (1973):173–178.

112. Magoffin, C. American Medical Review Research Center (AMRRC), Washington, DC Personal Communication, June 4, 1992.

113. Mansfield, E. *Statistics for Business and Economics: Methods and Applications.* New York: Norton, 1980.

114. Markert, R.J. Relationship of Old and New MCAT Scores to Performance on the Part III Examination of the NBME. *J. Med. Educ.* **60** (1985):53–55.

115. Markert, R.J. Cognitive Predictors of Residency Performance. *Resident Staff Physician* (August 1989):53–58.

116. Markson, L.E., Nash, D.B., Louis, D.Z., & Gonnella, J.S. Clinical Outcomes Management and Disease Staging. *Eval. Health Prof.* **14** (1991):201–227.

117. Marshall, J. Assessment of Problem-Solving Ability. *Med. Educ.* **11** (1977):329–334.

118. Marshall, J.R., & Fabb, W.E. The Construction of Patient Management Problems. Medical Education Booklet No 12. Dundee, Scotland: Association for the Study of Medical Education, 1981.

119. McCollister, R.J. The Use of Part I National Board Scores in the Selection of Residents in Ophthalmology and Otolaryngology. *JAMA* **259** (1988):240–242.

120. McGuire, C.H. Evaluation of Students and Practitioner Competence. In *Handbook of Health Professions Education*, C.H. McGuire,

R.P. Foley, A. Gorr & R.W. Richards, Eds., pp. 256–293. San Francisco: Jossey-Bass, 1983.

121. McGuire, C.H. Medical Problem-Solving: A Critique of the Literature. *J. Med. Educ.* **60** (1985):587–595.

122. McGuire, C.H. The Curriculum for the Year 2000. *Med. Educ.* **23** 91989):221–227.

123. Monk, M.A., & Thomas, C.B. Characteristics of Male Medical Students Related to Their Subsequent Careers. *Johns Hopkins Med. J.* **127** (1970):254–272.

124. Morton, J.B., & MacBeth, W.A.A.G. Correlation Between Staff, Peer, and Self Assessments of Fourth-Year Students in Surgery. *Med. Educ.* **11** (1977):167–170.

125. Mullen, B. *Advanced Basic Meta-Analysis*, Hillsdale, NJ: Lawrence Erlbaum, 1989.

126. Murden, R., Galloway, G.M., Reid, J.C., & Colwill, J.M. Academic and Personal Predictors of Clinical Success in Medical School. *J. Med. Educ.* **53** (1978):711–719.

127. Murdock, B.B. The Serial Position Effect on Recall. *J. Exp. Psychol.* **64** (1962):482–486.

128. Murphy, R.T. Ratings. In *Encyclopedia of Educational Evaluations*, S.B. Anderson, S. Ball & R.T. Murphy, Eds., pp. 315–319. San Francisco: Jossey-Bass, 1981.

129. Myers, C.J., Rubeck, R.F., & Meredith, K. An Investigation of Nonresponse Bias in Medical Students Assessment of Instruction. *Res. Higher Educ.* **19** (1983):461–467.

130. Neufeld, V.R., & Norman, G.R., Eds. *Assessing Clinical Competence.* New York: Springer, 1986.

131. Newble, D.I., & Swanson, D.B. Psychometric Characteristics of the Objective Structured Clinical Examination. *Med. Educ.* **22** (1988): 335–341.

132. Nie, N.H., Hull, C.H., Jenkins, J.G., Steinbrenner, K. & Bent, D.H. *SPSS: Statistical Package for the Social Sciences.* (2d ed.) New York: McGraw-Hill, 1975.

133. Norcini, J.J., Grosso, L.J., Shea, J.A., & Webster, G.D. The Relationship Between Features of Residency Training and ABIM Certifying Examination Performance. *J. Gen. Intern. Med.* **2** (1987):330–336.

134. Norcini, J.J., Webster, J.G., Grosso, I.J., Blank, L.L., & Benson, J.A. Ratings of Residents' Clinical Competence and Performance on Certification Examination. *J. Med. Educ.* **62** (1987):457–462.

135. O'Leary, D. S. Beyond Generic Occurrence Screening (Editorial). *JAMA* **265** (1991):1993–194.

136. Paiva, R.E.A. Reliability in Follow-up Evaluations of Graduates as Residents. *Proc. Annu. Conf. Res. Med. Educ.* **18** (1979):118–123.

137. Patel, V.L., Groen, G. J. & Norman, G.N. Effects of Conventional and Problem-based Medical Curricula on Problem Solving. *Acad.*

Med. **66** (1991):380–389.
138. Peters, A.S., & Schimpfhauser, F.T. Changes in Self-Evaluation During Third-year Clinical Rotations. *Proc. Annu. Conf. Res. Med. Educ.* **28** (1989):175–180.
139. Peterson, O., Andrews, L.P., Spain, R.S., & Greenberg, B.G. An Analytical Study of North Carolina General Practice. *J. Med. Educ.* **31** (Dec. 1956 Part 2) Suppl.
140. Petrusa, E.R., Blackwell, T.A., Rogers, L.P., Saydjari, C., Parcel, S., & Gukian, J.C., An Objective Measure of Clinical Performance. *Am. J. Med.* **83** (1987):34–42.
141. Petrusa, E.R., Blackwell, T.A., & Ainsworth, M.A. Reliability and Validity of an Objective Structured Clinical Examination for Assessing the Clinical Performance of Residents. *Arch. Intern. Med.* **150** (1990): 573–577.
142. Piel, G. Attributes of Excellence. *Sci. Amer.* **246** (1982):98–99.
143. Pisicano, N.J., Veloski, J.J., Brucker, P.C., & Gonnella, J.S. Classifying the Content of Board Certification Examinations. *Acad. Med.* **64** (1989):149–154.
144. Price, P.B., Taylor, C.W., Richards, J.M., & Jacobsen, T.L. Measurement of Physician Performance *J. Med. Educ.* **39** (1964):203–211.
145. Price, P.B., Taylor, C.W., Richards, J.M., & Jacobsen, T.L. *Measurement of Physician Performance: Final Report.* cooperative Research Program, Contract No. OE-2-10-093. Washington, DC: U.S. Office of Education, U.S. Department of Health, Education and Welfare, 1964.
146. Price, P.B. A Search for Excellence. *Am. J. Surg.* **118** (1969):815–821.
147. Price, P.B., Taylor C.W., Nelson, D.E., Lewis, E.G., Loughmiller, G.C., Mathiesen, R., Murray, S.L., & Maxwell, J.G. *Measurement and Predictors of Physician Performance: Two Decades of Intermittently Sustained Research.* Salt Lake City, UT: Aaron Press, 1973.
148. Rabinowitz, H.K., & Hojat, M. A Comparison of the Modified Essay Question and Multiple-choice Question Formats: Their Relationships to clinical Competence. *Fam. Med.* **5** (1989):364–367.
149. Ramsey, P.G., Carline, J.D., Inusi, T.S., Larson, E.B., Logerfo, J.P., Norcini, J.J., & Wenrich, M.D. Changes Over Time in the Knowledge Base of Practicing Internists. *JAMA*, **226** (1991):1103–1107.
150. Reinhardt, A.M., and Gray, R.M. A Social Psychological Study of Attitude Change in Physicians. *J. Med. Educ.* **47** (1972):112–117.
151. Render, G.F., & Jackson, H.D. Preveterinary Performance Admissions Criteria and Personality Variables as Predictors of Success in Veterinary School. *J. Vet. Educ.* **2** (1972):3-6.
152. Rethans, J.J., Sturmans, F., Drop, van der Vlueten, C. & Hobus, P. General Practice: Does Competence of General Practitioners Predict Their Performance? Comparison Between Examination Set-

ting and Actual Practice. *Br. Med. J.* **303** (1991):1377–1380.
153. Reynolds, H.N., Haupt, M.T., Thill–Baharozian, M.C., & Carlson, R.W. The Impact of Critical Care Physician Staffing on Patients with Septic Shock in a University Hospital Medical Intensive Care Unit. *JAMA* **260** (1988):3446–3450.
154. Reznick, R., et al. An Objective Structure Clinical Examination for the Licentiate: Report of the Pilot Project of the Medical Council of Canada. *Acad. Med.* **67** (1992):487–494.
155. Rich, E.C., Schlossberg, L., Luxenberg, M. & Korn, J. Influence of a Preventive Care Educational Intervention on Physician Knowledge, Attitudes, Beliefs, and Practice. *Prev. Med.* **18** (1989): 847–855.
156. Richards, J.M., Jr., Taylor, C.W., & Price, P.B. The Prediction of Medical Intern Performance. *J. Appl. Psychol.* **46** (1962):142–146.
157. Richardson, I.M. Examination Performance and the Future Career of Aberdeen Medical Graduates. *Med. Educ.* **14** (1980):356–359.
158. Roberts, J.S., Radany, M.H., & Nash, D.B. Privilege Delineation in a Demanding New Environment. *Ann. Intern. Med.* **108** (1988): 880–886.
159. Ronai, A.K., Golmon, M.E., Shanks, C.E., Schafer, M.F., & Brunner, E.A. Relationship Between Past Academic Performance and Results of Specialty In-Training Examinations. *J. Med. Educ.* **59** (1984): 341–344.
160. Rosenfeld, L.M., Hojat, M., Veloski, J.J., Blacklow, R.S. & Goepp, C.E. Delays in Completing Medical School: Predictors and Outcomes. *Teach. Learn. Med.* **4** (1992):162–167.
161. Rosenthal, R. *Meta-Analysis Procedures for Social Research.* Beverly Hills, CA: Sage, 1984.
162. Rothman, A.I., Cohen, R., Dirks, F.R., Poldre, P., & Ross, J. Validity and Reliability of a Domain-Referenced Test of Clinical Competence for Foreign Medical Graduates. *Acad. Med.* **66** (1991):423–427.
163. Rubin, H.R., Rogers, W.H., Kahn, K.L., Rubenstein, L.V., & Brook, R.H. Watching the Doctor Watchers: How Well Do Peer Review Organization Methods Detect Hospital Care Quality Problems? *JAMA* **267** (1992):2349–2354.
164. SAS Institute, Inc. *SAS User's Guide: Statistics* (5th ed.) Cary, North Carolina: SAS Institute Inc., 1985.
165. Schlackman, N. Integrating Quality Assessment and Physician Incentive Payment. (Editorial) *Qual. Rev. Bull* **15** (1989):234–237.
166. Schlackman, N. The Quality Care Cycle. *Qual. Rev. Bull.* **17** (1991): 360–364.
167. Schmidt, F.L., & Hunter, J.E. Development of a General Solution to the Problem of Validity Generalization. *J. Appl. Psychol.* **62** (1977):529–540.

168. Schroeder, S.A., & Kabcenell, A.I. Do Bad Outcomes Mean Substandard Care? (Editorial) *JAMA* **265** (1991):1995.
169. Seegal, D., & Wertheim, A.R. On the Failure to Supervise Students' Performance of Complete Physical Examination. *JAMA* **180** (1962): 476–477.
170. Spearman, C.E., *The Ability of Man*. New York: Macmillan, 1927.
171. Spellacy, W.N. The Use of National Board Scores in Selecting Residents for Obstetrics and Gynecology. *Am. J. Obstet. Gynecol.* **153** (1985):605–607.
172. Sperling, G. The information Available in Brief Visual Presentation. *Psychol. Monographs* **74** (1960) (Whole No. 498).
173. Stillman, P.L. Regan, M.B., Swanson, D.B., Case, S., McCahan, J., Feinblatt, J., Smith, S.R., Williams, J., & Nelson, D.V. An Assessment of the Clinical Skills of Fourth-year Students at Four New England Medical Schools. *Acad. Med.* **65** (1990):320–326.
174. Stillman, P., Regan, M.B., & Swanson, D. A Diagnostic Fourth Year Performance Assessment. *Arch. Intern. Med.* **19** (1987):1981–1985.
175. Taylor, C.R. Great Expectations: The Reading Habits of Year II Medical Students. *N. Engl. J. Med.* **326** (1992):1436–1440.
176. Taylor, C.W. Education, Developing Effectively Functioning People: The Accountable Goal of Multiple Talent Teaching. *Education* **94** (Nov.–Dec. 1973):99–110.
177. Taylor, C.W., & Ellison, R.L. Biographical Predictors of Scientific Performance. *Science* **155** (1967):1075–1080.
178. Taylor, C.W., & Ellison, R.L. Predicting Creative Performances from Multiple Measures. In *Widening Horizons in Creativity*, C.W. Taylor, Ed., pp. 245–258. New York: Wiley, 1964.
179. Taylor, C.W., Ghiselin, B., & Yagi, K. *Exploratory Research on Communication Abilities and Creative Abilities*. Final Report to U.S. Air Force under Grant AF-AFOSR 144–63 [available from author], 1967 (see pp. 144–163).
180. Thompson, W.G., Lipkin, M., Gilbert, D.A., Guzzo, R.A., & Roberson, L. Evaluating Evaluation: Assessment of the American Board of Internal Medicine Resident Evaluation Form. *J. Gen. Intern Med.* **5** (1990):214–217.
181. Thorndike, R.L. The Role of General Ability in Prediction. *J. Vocational Behav.* **29** (1986):332–339.
182. Tobachnik, B.G., & Fidell, L.S. *Using Multivariate Statistics*. New York: Harper & Row, 1983.
183. Tolnay, S. Continuing Medical Education and Career Choice Among Graduates of Problem-Based and Traditional Curricula. *Med. Educ.* **25** (1991):414–420.
184. Turner, B.J., Hojat, M., & Gonnella, J.S. Using Ratings of Resident Competence to Evaluate NBME Examination Passing Standards. *J. Med. Educ.* **62** (1987):572–581.

185. Tuteur, P.B. Internal Medicine Chief Residents Want Changes in Education. (Resident Forum). *JAMA* **264** (1990):175.

186. Veloski, J., Herman, M.W., Gonnella, J.S., Zeleznik, C., & Kellow, W.F. Relationship Between Performance in Medical School and First Postgraduate Year. *J. Med. Educ.* **54** (1979):909–916.

187. Veloski, J.J., Hojat, M., & Gonnella, J.S. A Validity Study of Part III of the National Board Examination. *Eval. Health Prof.* **13** (1990): 227–240.

188. Veloski, J.J., Rabinowitz, H.K., & Robeson, M.R. Cueing in Multiple Choice Questions: A Reliable, Valid Economical Solution. *Proc. Annu. Conf. Res. Med. Educ.* **27** (1988):195–200.

189. Verhulst, S.J., Colliver, J.A., Paiva, R.E.A., & Williams, R.G. A Factor Analysis Study of Performance of First-Year Residents. *J. Med. Educ.* **61** (1986):132–134.

190. Volle, R.L. Using National Board of Medical Examiners Scores in Selection of Residents. *JAMA* **259** (1988):266.

191. Vu, N.V., Barrows, H.S., Marcy, M.L., Verhulst, S.J., Colliver, J.A., & Travis, T.A. Six Years of Comprehensive, Clinical Performance-Based Assessment Using Standardized Patients at the Southern Illinois University School of Medicine. *Acad. Med.* **67** (1992):42–50.

192. Vu, N.V., Colliver, J.A., & Verhulst, S.J. Factor Structure of Clinical Competence as Assessed in a Performance-Based Examination Using Standardized Patients. In *Current Developments in Assessing Clinical Competence.* I.R. Hart, R.M. Harden, & J. DesMarchais, Eds., Montreal, PQ: Can-Heal Publications, 1992.

193. Wagoner, N.E. & Suriano, J.R. Recommendations for Changing the Residency Selection Process Based on a Survey of Program Directors. *J. Med. Educ.* **67** (1992):459–465.

194. Wagoner, N.E., Suriano, J.R., & Stoner, J.A. Factors Used by Program Directors to Select Residents. *J. Med. Educ.* **61** (1986):10–21.

195. Wakeford, R., & Roberts, S. Thirty Years on: Examination Performance and Career Success of the 1950–1 Intake of Cambridge Medical Students. *Br. Med. J.* **286** (1983):1796–1798.

196. Warrick, S.S., & Crumrine, R. S. Predictors of Success in an Anesthesiology Residency. *J. Med. Educ.* **61** (1986):591–595.

197. Weston, J.A., & Dubovsky, S.L. Evaluating Medical School Graduates of A Reduced Course Program: A Preliminary Report. *J. Med. Educ.* **59** (1984):1–16.

198. Williams, D.A. Personality and Vocational Choice. Ph.D. diss, University of Georgia, 1979 [Dissertation Abstracts International, 39(7-B),3493].

199. Williams, R.G., Barrow, H.S., Vu, N.V., Verhulst, S.J., Colliver, J.A., Marcy, M., & Steward, D. Direct, Standardized Assessment of Clinical Competence. *Med. Educ.* **21** (1987):482–489.

200. Williams, R.G., & Colliver, J.A. A Study of Errors Attributable to Use

of NBME Part I Scores for Residency Selection Purposes. *Proc. Annu. Conf. Res. Med. Educ.* **26** (1987):43–47.
201. Willoughby, T.L., & Bixby, A.R. Cross Validation of the Quarterly Profile Examination. *Educ. Psychol. Meas.* **51** (1991):691–697.
202. Wingard, J.R., & Williamson, J.W. Grades as Predictors of Physicians' Career Performance: an Evaluative Literature Review. *J. Med. Educ.* **48** (1973):311–322.
203. Woodward, C.A. Assessing the Relationship Between Medical Education and Subsequent Performance. *Assess. Eval. Higher Educ.* **9** (1984):19–29.
204. Woodward, C.A., & Dinham, S.M. Methodological Factors in Studying Medical Graduates. *Eval. Health Care Prof.* **5** (1982):95–111.
205. Wu, A.W., Folkman, S., McPhee, S.J., & Lo, B. Do House Officers Learn from Their Mistakes? *JAMA* **265** (1991):2089–2094.
206. Yindra, K.J., Rosenfeld, P.S., & Donnelly, M.B. Medical School Achievements as Predictors of Residency Performance. *J. Med. Educ.* **63** (1988):356–363.
207. Young, R.H. Medical Education in the United States. *J. Med. Educ.* **34** (1959):802–813.
208. Yufit, R.J., Pollack, G.H., & Waserman, E. Medical Specialty Choice and Personality. *Arch. Gen. Psychiat.* **20** (1969):89–99.
209. Zeleznik, C., Hojat, M., Goepp, C.E., Amadio, P., Kowlessar, O.D., & Borenstein, B.D. Measurement of Certainty in Medical School Examination: A Pilot Study on Noncognitive Dimensions of Test-Taking Behavior. *J. Med. Educ.* **63** (1988):881–891.
210. Zeleznik, C., Hojat, M., & Veloski, J. Levels of Recommendation for Students and Academic Performance in Medical School. *Psychol. Rep.* **52** (1983):851–858.
211. Zeleznik, C., Hojat, M., & Veloski, J. Long-Range Predictive and Differential Validities of the Scholastic Aptitude Test in Medical School. *Educ. Psychol. Meas.* **43** (1983):223–232.

References for Chapter 16

212. Liu, B.X., Mei, R.L., Niu, W.D., Zhang, Z., Qiu, X.X., & Wang, L. Predictive Validity of a National Examination for Medical Graduates in the People's Republic of China. *Academic Medicine* **65** (1990): 505–511.
213. Shaw, B. *Saint Joan*. New York: Penguin Books Inc. (1946).
214. Poincare, H. *The Foundations of Science*. Lancaster, PA: The Science Press (1946).
215. Carroll, L. *Through the looking glass*. New York: Bantam Classic (1983).

Index of Names

Index of Subjects